THE PHYSICIAN WELLNESS PROJECT

A Doctor's Roadmap to Job Satisfaction

Gregory Charlop, MD

Dr. Greg, LLC, Atlanta, Georgia

IMPORTANT DISCLAIMER

endorsement, approval, or affiliation with any such third-party entities, products, or services by Gregory Charlop, MD, Dr. Greg LLC, or its affiliates. Likewise, these third-party entities have not endorsed or approved this book or its contents. Any trademarks or registered trademarks mentioned within this book are the property of their respective owners.

By reading this book, you acknowledge that you have read, understood, and agreed to this disclaimer.

AUTHOR'S NOTE

Dear colleague,

Thank you for supporting a fellow doc. Like you, I'm trying to make the world a better place while enjoying quality time with family, hobbies, and self-care.

If you're a nurse, physician assistant, nurse practitioner, CRNA, or any working healthcare professional, thank you for joining us. Please note that while I use the term "physician" throughout the book, most of the content here applies to you as well. I'm devastated by the skyrocketing rate of nurse burnout and will do whatever I can to help.

After practicing medicine across the country, pursuing dream projects, being on TV, and raising two wonderful daughters, I am convinced we can find joy and balance in our careers.

I know you're busy, and I appreciate you sharing some time with me. I promise to make this worth your while. If you have any questions about my journey, contact me anytime at www.GregoryCharlopMD.com

I have loads of useful (and some goofy) videos on my YouTube page: https://www.youtube.com/@physicianwellnessproject   Let's   get   started!   Gregory Charlop, MD

Contents

Chapter 1

Introduction

If you had told me five or ten years ago that I would be able to work in medicine without taking call, working nights, holidays, or weekends, yet still be able to take care of patients and make more money, I would never have believed you. If you had told me that I would be able to take a vacation with my family whenever my kids were out of school, including during Thanksgiving and New Year's, and not have to compete with my colleagues in some crazy lottery for these few precious weeks, I would never have believed you. If you had told me that by now, I would've written four books, started multiple charity conferences to support girls' sports and women business leaders, that I would've traveled the world, started several businesses, and still had more time for the gym, I would've thought you'd lost it.

But that is where my life is today, and that is the position you'll be in once you're finished reading this book. I'm Dr. Greg. I will show you what you need to do to get more joy from medicine and more happiness out of your clinical career so you can better balance caring for patients with time for family and self-care like sleep, the gym, going out, or hobbies you enjoy. I'll show you how to make medicine work for you. Or if you want to leave medicine after we think it through together. I'll show you how to do that as well.

Back in 2019, I finally decided. I was going to do it. I got calls from family and friends, all thinking I had gone mad. Everybody asked me if I was sure I had made the right decision. Colleagues, medical school classmates, and anyone who knew me thought I might be making a grave mistake. My peers told me, "Just stay a few years longer. If you do, then you get free healthcare for life. You'll get a bigger pension and move up in the seniority ranks. Things will get better with time. Just stick around longer."

I have heard this for years, and I did stick around longer, but eventually, I did what nobody I knew had ever done. I decided to leave my long-term stable job with a hospital, a hospital that I loved. You see, I'm a pediatric anesthesiologist. And for most of my, at that time, 14-year career, I had worked full-time at a major tertiary hospital in California. Eventually, when I had kids, I realized that full-time was unsustainable, and I switched to part-time. First, I worked 80% time, and ultimately, I even made my way down to 60% time, which is quite rare and was rarely granted.

I loved seeing patients. I loved working and caring for others, including the less fortunate, who needed the care. I had tremendous respect for my colleagues, including the physicians and nurses. And honestly, I even admired the hospital administration. I thought everybody meant well. The problem was that I just wanted something different than they had to offer. And although I love patients, I honestly got tired of the call. Even when I was just 60% time and had fewer calls than many of my colleagues, I still couldn't do it.

You all know the feeling. We go to bed at night. If you are on pager call like I was, you would check your pager or your phone. You would check five or ten times to ensure the ringer was on, that you had reception, and that you hadn't missed anything before bed. You would try to go to sleep. Then, you would keep looking at your phone or your pager to see that you hadn't missed anything.

I never could get a good night's sleep because I was always worried I'd get called in. And you know how it is. When you're called in in the middle of the night, it would usually be some disastrous thing. That was tough.

I respect people who do it. I'm so thankful for them, but at that point, I realized I couldn't do it anymore. I'm not a night person. I never was. Even in high school, if I had a big assignment, I'd go to bed early the day before and get up early the next day. Nights are not my thing.

The holidays were tough, too. We'd work Thanksgiving or New Year's. Halloween was a big one. I remember when my kids were young. They would dress up in Halloween costumes; all they wanted to do was go trick-or-treating with me. And I wanted to go out with them. I admit I love Halloween myself. But I really loved seeing my kids dress up and go out, especially when they were little enough to want to be with me. I could see my kids growing up and having these fun holidays without me, and I couldn't take that anymore.

And finally, even though I respected and admired my coworkers, anytime you work with the same group of people for a long time, there's bound to be politics. It's just the nature of any kind of group like that. Although I doubt the politics where I worked were any worse than elsewhere, I didn't need it anymore. I was ready to move on and do my own thing.

Here's the deal. I fancy myself as a creative person. As a college student, I wasn't even sure I wanted to go into medicine because I liked doing so many other things.

I don't regret becoming a doctor. I'm thankful for it because I love the patients, and it was a fantastically stable job during economic turmoil. But I still like doing other stuff.

I had fun with real estate. I flipped homes. I started a real estate syndicate. I had rental properties. I even started some real estate technology conferences and wrote a book about real estate technology, which you would not expect to do in clinical medicine. I had podcasts. I did all these different sorts of things. But the problem was, I realized I didn't have enough in the tank to do all that stuff, plus do call, nights, weekends, and holidays. I didn't have it in me.

So I left. I left my hospital, and I left without a plan.

I didn't know what I was going to do. I just knew that I wanted to take control of my schedule. I wanted to retake control of my life. I wanted to sleep at night without worrying about being called in, and I wanted to have the opportunity to explore my other interests. So I left.

We moved, and I started doing different clinical experiences I hadn't tried before. I did pediatric dental procedures in dentists' offices. We had these portable anesthesia machines, and we had these tackle boxes worth of drugs. It was cool, and it was different.

I worked in Beverly Hills with some of the world's top plastic surgeons. I traveled all over the country and did all kinds of neat stuff. I even tried telemedicine, which was a lot of fun.

The best part - I didn't have call or nights. I didn't have the office politics that I had before. And I could be with my kids whenever they needed me. And I had time for other projects like philanthropic conferences and writing books.

Plus,

I was on TV! How cool is that for a humble physician?!

That brings me to the point of this book: I want to help you. I want to help fellow doctors and other healthcare professionals get more joy out of medicine. I want to make it so you can do some of the same things that I did or different things that are more fun or better than I've done. I want to help you reconfigure your career so you love what you're doing and have time for your family and kids, activities, hobbies, sleep, the gym, sports, or whatever you like to do.

In addition to my clinical medicine practice, I enjoy one-on-one consulting with physicians or other healthcare professionals looking to improve their lives and get more joy out of their practice. I offer online courses for healthcare professionals (like you!) looking to make a change and have some fun.

I've talked to a lot of physicians. So many of us are suffering. We're suffering from the hours and the call, but we're also struggling with moral injury. We went into medicine to care for patients, but due to factors beyond our control like bureaucracy, excessive administration, billing and compensation practices, and compliance, doctors feel that they're no longer spending their time doing what they went into medicine for, caring for patients. Instead of the joy we hope to get out of being with others in trying times, many of us feel we're battling administrators, insurance companies, or mid-level management. There's a loss of autonomy for physicians.

As a result of this moral injury and physician burnout, people are having a hard time continuing. Physician burnout, which may affect you and your colleagues, is a serious problem for your mental and physical health, job satisfaction, and society at large. It's vital for us to keep doctors happy and productive, and to empower doctors to make a difference in the lives of our patients without feeling like everything is a struggle.

If you're a physician or any healthcare provider who is feeling burnt out from clinical medicine, if you've lost your joy and you want to rekindle that energy, or if you're considering switching careers altogether and you want to know what it's like, this book is for you. This is your roadmap.

You deserve to be happy. You deserve to love your job. You deserve to love taking care of patients. You deserve to look forward to getting up in the morning and going to work or doing whatever you choose to do with your day. You worked so hard for this, and you earned it. You earned the right to enjoy time with your family, your children, your spouse, your siblings, your parents, and your friends. You deserve time to do your hobbies and to contribute to society. You earned this. You could do this.

Together, let's get started.

Chapter 2

Job Dissatisfaction, the Medical School Paradox, and a Bucket of Crabs

The Medical School Paradox

I'll date myself here and tell you I went to school before the internet era kicked in. For those of you of my vintage, you may remember that near checkout stands at many stores, in electronic stores, for example, they would have a rack of inexpensive software you could buy.

They had games, simple productivity tools, gardening tips, recipes, and the like. They were all inexpensive, impulse buy kind of things.

I saw this and thought it would be a great opportunity to sell first-person games, where you have a character and move through a maze, exploring.

I don't know how to program, but I loved the potential. I thought, *How great would it be to build a game where you had a fantasy character, explored a maze in a castle, and played it for a couple of hours? It'd be an easy sale for a couple of dollars.*

As a college student, I created a company to sell these games. I found programmers since I didn't know how to program. I found artists since I was terrible at art. And together, we created some software.

While I was a student at UCLA, I did all kinds of fun, creative activities like that. There were a lot of underserved people near our Los Angeles campus that needed help. They had high blood pressure or other chronic medical problems but didn't know what to do about it. They were undertreated.

So, we created a series of health fairs. Together with my peers, we got the support of different organizations to fund this, including, believe it or not, an MCAT test prep company. They gave us some money.

We brought people into a community center. We measured their blood pressure and heart rate and gave them simple health questionnaires. We even had some referrals to free clinics for them.

We were just college students. We couldn't diagnose or treat anything, but we knew there were many untreated problems. We brought people from the community together and sent them to places where they could get care for their chronic medical conditions. And this was great. I felt good about it and knew we made a difference.

As a high school and early college student, I loved debate. We traveled around to debate tournaments. It was fun trying to destroy other people on the stage.

I did all this while attending school, getting good grades, and taking advanced classes to get into medical school. I tell you this not because there's anything special about what I did. You did just as many exciting extracurriculars as I did.

Many of my peers did mindblowing things with international development projects and philanthropy. So many great premed artists painted beautiful pieces or made mind-blowing sculptures. My peers were learning four or five languages. They were mentoring. I've known many people in medical school who mentored underserved children when they were in college. They would go into schools or create a mentorship program to help kids succeed when otherwise they would've been left behind.

I've known people in medical school who, while in college and high school, set up and ran animal shelters or launched monumental projects with their religious groups to help people in need.

I'm jealous of the people in medical school I knew who were professional chefs. They were so good that they cooked at restaurants. Some even had careers as chefs, left those jobs, and went into medical school.

Some folks played elite sports. I've known several people who were top-flight basketball, volleyball, or baseball players, swimmers, golfers, or tennis players.

My medical school colleagues did all these fantastic things in high school and college. Why? They were creative people who didn't want to just go to class. They wanted more. They had the itch to start organizations, become the best at something, or help others.

And they also did it partly because this is what medical schools expect of the people they accept. That's great. I support it. It is terrific that medical schools look at grades, test scores, and life experiences.

What have you started? Whom have you helped? What are your talents? What adversity have you overcome to be a doctor?

I admire you.

We want our physicians to be more than just school nerds. We want your physicians to be well-rounded people who care, have overcome adversity, and enjoy varied interests.

But here's where the problem lies, as many of you will relate. You're taking all these people with all these interests, that started organizations, that were elite athletes, that were top musicians, or that traveled internationally to help underserved communities, and you shove them through medical school, residency, and fellowship. Now, they're in a career that consumes 60 hours a week and all their working time. You've taken people with diverse, varied interests and put them in a career that snuffs out those interests.

Medical schools say, "I want people who started companies or clubs, who traveled internationally to help, who devoted an inordinate amount of time to perfecting their tennis game to come." But once you're done with medical school, you won't be able to do any of those things because your career is so demanding. And when you're not working, if you're lucky, you'll have a little bit of time to go to the gym and see your family, and that's about it.

This medical school paradox is a significant source of dissatisfaction because you take creative people with creative entrepreneurial drive, drives for excellence in crafts and sports, art, and music, but then you don't let them do any of those things after training them.

The Long Runway

You had to work hard in high school to get into medical school. You clobbered yourself in high school because you needed good grades to get into an elite college - because you wanted to go to medical school.

You went to college and worked hard to get into medical school. You worked hard to earn good grades and took the college's most brutal courses. You took advanced organic chemistry, biochemistry, physics, and math classes. You may have taken extra language classes, the classics, or economics. You did all these things because you wanted to get into medical school. This took a lot of your time.

Okay, so you finally got into medical school. I don't have to tell any of you that medical school was hard. You had long hours of class. You had to go to preceptors and to doctor's offices across town. You worked late in the hospital. Perhaps for the first time, you were seeing sick patients. You might've even watched patients deteriorate or die under your team's care. That is hard. It's emotionally draining. It's time-consuming.

After attending (and possibly paying for) high school, college, and medical school, you now go to residency and, perhaps, fellowship. You're finally making some money, but much less than your peers. Many residents work 80 hours a week or more. Many residents take call. They work overnight, they work on weekends. The tremendous dedication one has to make to residency precludes most other fun activities.

You've finished your residency or fellowship. You've finally made it. You've finally reached your goal after all that hard work in high school, college, medical school, residency, and perhaps fellowship. You are a practicing physician.

Being a physician is one of the most rewarding and challenging jobs one could have. After all, how many other jobs give you such a tremendous opportunity to help people in need? But being a physician is challenging and takes a lot of time.

You put in all this time to get where you are. And now that you're *there*, you have to put in a lot more time to keep doing it. It feels like it never ends.

What were your friends doing while you were spending all this time on work? What were your peers in high school doing when you were taking all those AP classes? They were out having fun. What were your peers doing in college when you were starting companies, mastering the violin, and taking advanced mathematics classes? They were going out. They were going on dates; they were doing social things. They were having these adventures you couldn't because you were so busy with school.

What were your friends doing when you were a resident, making little money and working a lot? While you were overnight at the hospital, your friends were going out, getting married, and traveling the world. And your friends were probably making more money than you were. Throughout your training, you worked harder while making less money than most of your peers.

There are some professions, like investment banking, where people work hard in college. They may get an MBA. But, few people say that business school is nearly as demanding as medical school and residency. And yes, investment bankers, consultants, and lawyers work a lot. They pay their dues for a few years and then make so much money they can retire. If you've met investment bankers, many of those folks had much more fun in college than most of us docs.

I want to add an extra wrinkle to this: not only time and work, but you've sacrificed where you live. Most of us went to school not necessarily where we wanted to be but rather the best school we could get into that met our needs for going on to medical school and then residency. We went to residency and fellowship, not where we wanted to live, but where we were accepted. And many of you, particularly those in subspecialties, spent many years in a place you don't want to be.

For example, if you are a neuro ICU doctor and your passion is to take care of patients who have suffered brain trauma or hemorrhages, there aren't a lot of places in the country where you could train.

You might have wished to stay in California, Florida, or Boston. But if there wasn't a job or training program there, you would have to move clear across the country.

What about student loans? Many of you did not come from affluent families. You had to borrow money to go to college. And if you went to an elite private school, you probably had to borrow a lot. If you're a more recent grad, even if you went to a state school, you may have had to borrow a significant amount of money to be able to afford college. I don't have to tell you how expensive medical school is!

Finally, when you're working as a resident or fellow, while you do get some money, most people don't earn enough to start paying back student loans. The student loans you accumulated during college and medical school grow while you are in residency and fellowship. Once you've come out of all of this, you may have a substantial debt hanging over you, debt that you have to pay back.

When you combine all of this, you have the runway problem. You devoted much time to college, medical school, residency, and fellowship. You've done a lot of work. You have lived perhaps where you have not wanted to live to go to the schools or programs you needed. If you have a narrow specialty, you still might not be where you'd like to live. Your friends did all those fun things you didn't do because you were so busy training. And now you have an enormous student debt.

In other words, you may have done all this work because you wanted to become, for example, a pediatric endocrinologist. You went to medical school; you went to pediatric residency; you went into an endocrinology fellowship; you lived where you didn't want to live, and you worked hard.

What happens if, when you're done, you're either so limited in where you can live that you're not happy with those choices or don't like pediatric endocrinology anymore? (Note: No offense to pediatric endocrinologists; I'm just using you as an example!).

But if you've done all this, and you're living where you don't want to live and don't like the specialty anymore, you may feel stuck because of this long runway. You've put so much time and effort into becoming your specialty, a pediatric endocrinologist, that it almost feels impossible to do anything else.

The Treadmill Problem

I confess that I poached this concept from one of my favorite books, *The 4-Hour Workweek* by Tim Ferriss. If you haven't read this book, please consider checking it out. Yes, I know it's a few years old, but that book profoundly impacted me. It helped me reframe how I looked at things like work and time commitments to careers. It was eye-opening, and I recommend it to all the physicians I work with.

One of the things that Ferriss talks about is the treadmill. Here's how it works. Imagine you're at the gym, getting ready for a tough workout. You're sporting your grey sweats. You fill up your water bottle and hit the treadmill. You get on and start running. At first, it's moving slowly, and you have time to space out. You have time to look around the room. You might watch the gym's TV or catch up on a few text messages.

But you're committed to exercise and won't do a half-hearted workout. You start turning up the speed of the treadmill. You run faster and faster. You're getting in a good sweat. Because you're running fast now, you're not able to do the ancillary stuff you were doing before.

You can't watch *Star Trek*. You definitely can't concentrate enough to text your sister. You're undoubtedly unable to plan that weekend get-together with friends because you are too focused on staying on the treadmill. The treadmill's going fast, and if you get distracted, if you look too much to the left or the right, you'll fall. So you keep running on the treadmill. Forward.

Life in medicine can often be like that. You get going on the treadmill early in college. In medical school, then in residency, it ramps up. Now you're an attending. You are the one responsible for lives. You are the one who's on call. If you don't show up in the ER, for surgery, or at the clinic, there isn't anyone to replace you. You're running on the treadmill.

You're running on the treadmill and don't see what's passing you by. You're running on the treadmill and miss time with your best friends. They're taking a trip somewhere. You aren't going. They go out to lunch every Tuesday afternoon. You can't make it. You're running on the treadmill, and you give up your hobbies. You used to play violin; you used to play racquetball. No time for that now. You're running on the treadmill.

You do manage to get married. Now you have a spouse, but you're running on the treadmill. You don't have time to see your spouse because you're so busy trying to stay on target.

You're fortunate enough to have kids, but you don't see your kids. You'll fall off the treadmill if you turn to the left or right. You're running on the treadmill. You don't see them. Your kids are growing up, and you keep running on the treadmill.

You make accommodations to make this possible. You have nannies. You're changing your schedule. You are giving up your favorite activities. You're running on the treadmill.

You live where you don't want to live because of the demands of your specialty. *I'll move later*, you tell yourself. Once a job opens up in the city of your choice, you'll go there. But you're running on the treadmill.

All of that passes you by. Your life adjusts. You get used to what you're doing. You get used to the scenery passing you by and stay focused on one thing: staying upright and not falling over.

Eventually, after running on the treadmill for so long, you get beat. That extra water isn't doing anything for you. You're tired. You shut the machine off, and you look around.

If you're anything like me, you might think, *What was I doing on the treadmill this long, or how was I even able to stay here? What did I miss?*

You think, *What have I done? What was I doing? While I was here running but not going anywhere, I missed time with my best friends. I forgot my hobbies. I surrendered my sports. I lost time with my spouse, and my kids are all grown up. All that passed me by because I couldn't look to the left. I couldn't look to the right. I just needed to keep on running forward but in place.*

What keeps us on the treadmill? Well, part of it is its own momentum. You've been doing it for a long time. You've been running it for a while. It's picking up steam. You feel like you can't afford to fall off.

You're also bought off. This is an idea that Tim Ferriss mentions in The 4-Hour Workweek. Your company, medical group, or hospital can buy you off to keep you on the treadmill. They may give you a vacation here or there. Occasionally, you'll get a cruise or something, just enough to keep you feeling like it's worth it. Just enough to prevent you from looking elsewhere.

You might get a small bonus or a raise. You might make extra money to keep you on the treadmill. This one works for me; you might get an occasional free lunch. You feel so great about that free lunch you keep running without going anywhere. It's incredible how much we will give up for that free lunch.

The Crab Problem

I know you were waiting for this one. I want to tell you a little story that I heard somewhere. I can't remember where I heard it.

I must tell you, I don't even know if this parable is true. For those who like research, please don't fact-check me on it. Or if you do, send me a message. I want to find out what you learn.

But here's the story. Fishermen go out, and they catch crabs. They put the crabs, live crabs, in a bucket. I'm from San Francisco, so I saw lots of these crabs.

They put the crabs in the bucket. They're alive; they're wiggling around; they're moving. They're doing everything. But the fishermen don't need to put a lid on the bucket. Why don't they need to do that? Why don't they cover the bucket to prevent the crabs from escaping?

Well, it turns out that when one crab tries to climb out of the bucket to escape, the other crabs reach up and pull that crab back down into the bucket. In a sense, the crabs in the bucket act as the jail wardens for each other, keeping all of them stuck. Ultimately, at least in the crabs' case, they keep themselves trapped till they're doomed.

Most of my physician clients and I had this problem. You'll see the same phenomenon if someone is thinking about going part-time or leaving their medical group and going somewhere else. In other words, there's this crazy cultural crab-like behavior that discourages anyone from making a radical shift in their clinical medical career. Have you experienced it?

And a lot of the time, this can come from well-meaning people. You tell your colleagues, "I'm thinking about leaving medicine and becoming a writer." Or, "I'm considering leaving medicine to become a consultant." And you hear, "You can't do that. You've invested so much time to become a doctor. Writers don't make money. You won't be happy being a consultant. Your true calling is seeing patients in the clinic." You say to your colleagues, "I'm thinking about working part-time," and they'll tell you, "You can't do that. If you work part-time, you won't make enough money, and you'll never be able to retire. You won't be able to afford your house, or your kids won't be able to go to college."

Sometimes, colleagues will say things like this because they are genuinely concerned. Since they're uncomfortable with change, they feel you should be uncomfortable too. Or they think that because they need the money for their expensive house, you need it as well.

Perhaps they have a misconception about finances and don't realize that you have more money than you need. Because they are afraid, they spread that fear onto you.

Other times, your colleagues may be more like crabs and are jealous that you're considering escaping to do something else. Perhaps they've always wanted to do it but never had the courage, or their life wouldn't allow it. Or maybe they're worried that if you leave, they'll have more call or trouble replacing you. Everybody's different; every situation's different. But regardless, well-meaning or not, your colleagues will often try to discourage you from escaping.

Friends and family are often the same way. No, I don't think they're jealous of you, and I do believe your friends and family want the best for you. But they don't understand what life is like for you in your clinical career. Your lawyer, accountant, or musician buddies aren't experiencing your day-to-day life of a doctor.

All they know is that you spent so much time training to be a physician. They know you put so much effort into it. Perhaps they've known you from college or before and saw you struggling with your organic chemistry classes, the MCATs, and your applications. And they naturally assume that you should be doing this forever because you put all the time into it. But they don't understand the moral injury, demands, and unpredictability of the day that can wear us down.

And even the most well-meaning people, your friends and parents, may discourage you from leaving medicine. One legitimate comment they often make is, "How do you know if you leave, you'll succeed in what else you try? You're succeeding as a doctor; you're seeing patients; you're making a difference, and you're making an income. If you give that up and decide to become a sailor, speaker, lawyer, or something very different, there is no guarantee of success."

That is true, but that is a risk you must decide if you are willing to take. We'll cover this elsewhere in the book, but that risk is smaller than you think because there are backup plans. If you play your cards right, you could always return to medicine. Or if your first alternative career doesn't work, there are always other ones.

My point is not that you should ignore your colleagues, friends, or family. You should indeed listen to them. They may have unique insight into you or your situation or even know something about the alternative career you're considering.

Listen to them, but don't feel you need to please them. Because at the end of the day, this is your life. You have only one, and you need to make the decision that makes the most sense for you.

Chapter 3

Do Your Research

I hope I've convinced you that improving your career is possible. But you're probably feeling nervous. After all, there are critical decisions. That's why we need to do some research before jumping into anything.

I recommend everyone speak to a wealth management advisor or consultant.

Allow me to take a quick detour. There is a great book that I read: *Die with Zero*. I'm not doing the book justice in my summary, but there are two critical parts of *Die with Zero* that really affected me and could also speak to you.

The first one is that many of us over-save, and we leave money on the table when we die. In other words, we work too much; we make a lot of money, which goes into our bank accounts, investments, or property, and we save it for a rainy day. But we have too much in these accounts. And by the time we move on, we die with lots of money in our bank account, extra investments, cash, and other material goods.

It's tragic because we did all this extra work but got nothing from it. We worked all those long hours at the hospital; we toiled overnight; we got paid for it, but that money did nothing for us because we didn't use it.

In an ideal world, the moment we die, our bank account would have $0. We should spend our dough before we die.

I know what you're saying. "I don't want to use all my money for myself. I want to give some money to my family or charities." You absolutely should. But if you're going to give some money to your kids, or your spouse, or your favorite charity, you could do that *while you're alive*. Establish a trust and make those donations now to benefit the charity. Let your kids or family plan around it. You don't need to wait until you're dead to donate. Make those plans now; the money left over is yours, and you get to spend it as you wish.

You're also probably saying, "Well, if I plan on dying with zero but overshoot the wrong way and I spend too much money, that's a problem." That's where the financial planner comes in. I'll explain more in a moment.

The second part of *Die with Zero* is that we put off too many of our goals till later in life, and then we miss the window of opportunity where we could actually live our dreams.

Let me give you a silly example, but it makes sense. Say you've always wanted to skydive. When you were a 20-year-old, that was your big dream. You really wanted to jump out of (a perfectly good) airplane. But you put it off. You didn't have the time or money and were too focused on other things. Now you're 70. You may still want a skydive, but it's tough for a 70-year-old. In fact, it's probably not such a great idea. You've waited too long and missed your window of opportunity to parachute.

You want to spend time with your kids. You've got this window of time where your kids are home with you. They've got time and want to be with you. They haven't yet run off to college or start a family. But you're focused on other endeavors. You wait too long, and you miss your chance.

The upshot is that when we wait too long to do stuff that matters, those opportunities vanish.

That leads us to this issue of wealth management. Here's the deal. When you go to a wealth manager or financial planner, they consider your assets, liabilities, risks, lifestyle, health, and when you want to retire. They evaluate the relevant issues and say, "Are you in good shape?" They answer the question, "Do you need more money, or do you have too much?" And they give you an objective view of this.

I recommend this to all my physician consulting clients. I want doctors to speak to a financial planner to understand where they stand.

You want an independent financial planner. Ideally, I recommend going to someone who charges a flat fee, gives you their advice, and that's it. They're done with you. That way, their opinions are not tainted by their desire to sell you stocks or some other investment. You're retaining them for their opinion about where you are today. They know that they gain nothing by being dishonest, and you walk away feeling good with the answer they gave you.

Let me talk more about how these wealth management firms work. The first thing they'll do is take a look at your assets. Assets could be things like your savings and investments. They'll examine your properties and how much you have saved in home equity. They'll help you value your business.

Financial management professionals will look at your alternative income streams. For example, you may have money from book revenue or consulting. Perhaps you're collecting a pension or alimony. The wealth management people will look at that. The next thing is they'll take a look at costs. This is where they're invaluable.

They'll first consider your costs and these out in the future. They've got formulas and algorithms for this.

For example, there are some costs like insurance. You need life insurance. You need vehicle insurance. You need medical insurance. If you're leaving a W-2 job, you must buy your own. You'll need malpractice insurance. Your employer may provide that now, but you'll need it in the future unless you decide to leave medicine altogether. If you choose to leave medicine, you'll need to purchase a policy with a tail.

You may want to consider disability and long-term care insurance. Both can make sense, depending on your situation. You'll want to speak to your financial planner about them.

Some of you may encounter alimony or child support expenses, and you want to game these out.

There are some big-ticket expenditures unique to your situation that you'll want to consider. Your financial planner could help you determine how much you need to save.

A big one is children. Anyone with kids (I've got a couple of my own) knows how expensive children are. You want to think about things like their college costs. Are you going to save up money for them? How much do you need to save? Consider whether you need to save money for them to go to a state school or a more expensive, more prestigious private school. What about grad school?

Do your kids have special needs? They may need some extra financial assistance. You need to budget for that. Perhaps your kids are young now, but as they get older, you might want them to play baseball, golf, or tennis. Those are expensive activities; you'll need to save up for lessons and travel.

If you have a spouse, you'll want to consider your spouse's needs and save money to support them as necessary. If your parents or relatives depend on you, consider how you'll care for them. For example, if you have elderly parents or a sister or brother with special needs, you may need to budget some money to care for these folks.

Future moves are another big one, and this mistake snags many of us. I admit that tripped me up several times. Let me give you an example.

Let's say you love where you live, and it is affordable. Perhaps you own a condo. Everything is great, and you're happy because you have a short commute to work and you know your neighbors. It's perfect. But the area doesn't have such a great school district.

You don't have kids yet, but you plan to later. Perhaps you've got toddlers and are not yet worried about school. Eventually, you might need to move out of the low-cost area you're in now to a pricier neighborhood with better schools.

I encountered this when we moved from the Bay Area to Los Angeles. I thought, "Well, Los Angeles will be so much cheaper because everybody tells me how expensive the San Francisco Bay Area is."

But then we discovered that only a few pockets of Los Angeles have good schools. And if you want to live in those places, it costs you an arm and a leg.

While you may not be on the cusp of moving, you need to consider whether you'll need to move in the not-too-distant future for kids or for some other reason. Perhaps your spouse doesn't like where you're living. Or you'll want to change the scene. You might be living inland and you've always wanted to live by the beach. Living by the beach will cost more money. You may want to move in the future for many reasons, and you'll want to budget for that.

You want money you can easily access if you need to buy something in an emergency (i.e., a new roof). You'll also want reserve funds in case you have a prolonged period where you don't have an income.

If you're trying to launch a new business, for example, having money in the bank is essential so you don't feel pressured to stop prematurely.

In other words, say you want to start a company or charity and leave your clinical job. You're devoting all your time to your company. You saved some money, but three months have gone by, then four months have gone by. Your business has yet to take off, which is not surprising.

You don't want to feel you have to abandon your startup because you're worried that next month you won't be able to put food on the table or you won't be able to cover your kids' basketball camp.

At the same time, you want to avoid a fire-sale liquidation of your long-term portfolio positions. Doing so can result in potential massive investment losses or unplanned capital gains taxes.

That's how people lose big on investments. Someone buys stock or an expensive property while holding paltry savings. Then, they experience a large, unplanned expense. Next thing they know, they're desperate for money. They sell their assets at an inopportune time, and now they're stuck with a huge loss or a high tax bill. This isn't the position you want to be in. You can avoid this problem with an adequate rainy-day fund.

Another thing that financial planners can do is help you budget for big-ticket discretionary items in the future. You may want to take an expensive vacation across Australia or build a wine bar in your basement. Maybe your car is getting a little long in the tooth, and you want to get a flying electric car (they're coming!). Or you want a self-driving car for your teenage son. You'll need to save money for that.

There is likely stuff that you and I have yet to think of. A financial planner could help you figure that out. They can review a list and say, "Well, did you consider these things? You should save money for them."

Financial planners can assist you with tax planning and estate management. They could help you determine what you should do with your investments and how to fund your retirement. If you're starting a business, they can recommend a corporate structure that yields the greatest tax benefits.

And if you're looking at things like inheritance for your kids, or your spouse, or a charity, the sooner you speak to a financial planner, the sooner you can structure these things to get the best bang for your buck, which is going to matter because then, you don't have to work as much now.

If you're considering a career change, or even if you're kicking the tires, I strongly recommend you speak to a wealth management professional. Doctor's orders. You'll feel better afterward.

And here's the real zinger. Your finance pro may say, "Look, you have so much money saved up; if you retired today and never worked again, you'll be fine." How good would it feel to hear that? How liberating would it be to know that you have saved enough that, at this point in your life, everything is good, everything else is gravy?

Now, you can go and do what you want and not worry that you'll end up on the streets or be forced into a job you don't want out of financial desperation.

Or they may tell you, "You've got to work two or three more years, and then you're golden," and that's great. You plan around it. There's an end in sight. Or they may tell you the opposite. They may say, "You've got kids coming up. You've got these bills. You need to make more money to live the lifestyle you expect."

You may not want to hear that, but that is valuable information. You could plan around it and use that to decide, "Well, maybe cutting back my hours isn't such a good idea now. Maybe I need to work more." Ugh! But, better to know.

I hope I've convinced you to speak to a wealth advisor or financial planner. Thank me later.

With that in mind, we can move to the more fun and important question: what do you want to do with your life? What do you want to be when you grow up?

The question is, do you like clinical medicine? In other words, do you enjoy caring for patients but want to make some changes (perhaps a different location or work schedule)? Or do you want something entirely different and non-clinical? In other words, would you stay in medicine if you could make some modifications, or are you convinced it's time to kiss medicine goodbye and move on?

To make a sensible decision, you must first determine what's bothering you. That is going to take some time. If you still need to nail down what makes you unhappy with work, now's the moment for some hard-core reflection. Find inspiring places, whether in the shower, in a sauna, talking to your spouse, on a walk, or brainstorming on notepads (I like this one), and review what makes you happy and unhappy at work. I like to use a pad and write things down.

In my physician consulting practice, I am a sounding board for my clients. We have fun going back and forth, openly considering the plusses and minuses of every facet of a clinical job. When we're done, docs feel like a weight is lifted and enjoy greater clarity.

I need you to sit down and figure out what's bothering you. You should be more specific than some vague sense that you're unhappy with your career and would like to do something else.

I've worked with many physicians who are dissatisfied with their careers. Physicians are often bothered by a lack of time with kids. This is a big one. Your kids are growing up, and you don't see them. You're missing their soccer games. You miss their first day of school. You're not around to take them to their doctor's visits or to be there when they win the spelling bee.

You may not be able to be with your spouse as much as you want to. Or you feel like you are dumping everything on your spouse because you are constantly at work, and your spouse has to take care of everything. Or you're leaving everything to a nanny, relative, or an extended after-school program. They're raising your kids for you because you're constantly at work.

Call is tough. There's the direct impact of call on your schedule (and sleep). But there's also the psychological burden due to loss of control and the risk that something heinous will happen overnight.

I remember when I took call. I haven't taken call in years. But when I did, I'd go to bed, turn out the light, and check my phone or pager 50 times to ensure it was working and the ringer was on so I could be reached. And I would never really be able to sleep well because I always knew there was a chance that I would be called in.

When I was called in, it was for something disastrous in the middle of the night. I could never get a good night's rest. I was always on edge. Even if I had never been called in, the fear took its toll.

Administrators are another problem for many doctors. I've spoken to physicians nationwide who feel their relationship with hospital administration could be better. They suspect that the administrators aren't listening to them. They don't take their concerns seriously. Many doctors rightfully view themselves as the people bringing business into the hospital and making the hospital money, yet they feel that they have no authority within the hospital. That's because the administrators decide key issues rather than the physicians. This sense of powerlessness and bureaucracy can be quite crippling and painful.

Some people may want to leave because they dislike local politics. Some folks don't like the politics. If you've worked with the same group of doctors or nurses for a while, folks inevitably get on each other's nerves.

Maybe you're frustrated that you miss holidays or vacations due to your clinical responsibilities. When I was an anesthesiologist at a large hospital, we had a vacation lottery. People could rank the weeks they wanted off from one to ten.

Needless to say, everybody who had kids wanted the same weeks off – Thanksgiving, Christmas, New Year's, spring break, and a good part of the summer.

But since only so many people could be gone at once, most people wouldn't get what they wanted. Most people who wanted to be off for Thanksgiving would still be working Thanksgiving week, whereas their spouses and kids were off. And this was very dissatisfying for a lot of people.

I understand why this had to happen. But as the person on the receiving end being told you can't be off for Thanksgiving, it can be difficult. And I understand it from having dealt with that myself.

A lot of physicians also feel disrespected by the hospital, or perhaps by the nurses, colleagues, and even increasingly by patients. From what I understand, patients 15 years ago interacted with doctors differently than today. Many patients feel like they are experts because they've looked up something on Google. Dr. Google said one thing, and you say something else. What do you know, and how do you know more than their internet search?

Most of us are happy that our patients are taking some initiative and they're learning about their illnesses. I know I am. But it can be difficult when the patient thinks you don't know what you're talking about.

Many doctors are considering leaving medicine due to moral injury. We've discussed this elsewhere in the book, and it's a major reason people exit clinical medicine altogether.

As we covered earlier, moral injury is when your daily work, ethics, and values don't match your vision of how things would be. For example, you may be an obstetrician who went into medicine believing you would help mothers and deliver babies. Those are noble goals.

Here's the trouble. These idealistic young doctors see situations where people are coming in who didn't have prenatal care, who aren't doing what they should be doing to take care of their babies, and who are not listening to your advice. Or the hospital doesn't allow you to do what you feel is necessary to care for your patients. You suffer from moral injury.

These are some of the common reasons people want to leave medicine. Which of these, or all of them, is particularly causing your discomfort with your clinical career? Be honest. Be honest with yourself. Be honest with me and really think it through.

People sometimes leave medicine because they have no choice. It could be because of an illness or a physical limitation. For example, you or a family member has a medical condition preventing you from practicing medicine. If a child, spouse, parent, or sibling needs a lot of your attention, you may need to be with them instead of at work.

You may have issues with your medical license. Some readers may have lost their licenses due to lawsuits or diversion. If you have any of these restraints, you're likely looking for a career outside of medicine. But you want to retain the value you have from your medical degree. In other words, you may not be practicing medicine anymore, but you still want to get some mileage out of your doctor title.

I've just explored reasons why you may want to leave medicine. But I'd like you to be open-minded about this. Think of the things you like about what you are doing now.

What do you like about your medical practice? Be honest; be fair. I'm trusting you on this to give it some serious thought. Do you like your colleagues? Do you love your patients? Do you love the fact that you can help people in need? Do you like your work environment? Do you like dealing with high-pressure situations or complexity? Do you like feeling that you are making a difference?

You can be honest here. Do you like the income? Doctors are paid quite well, and it's fair to say that you're happy with that. Do you like the job stability? Doctors enjoy greater job stability and dependability than most other professions because doctors are in short supply, at least in the foreseeable future.

So think. What do you like about what you're doing now? Even if you're considering leaving medicine, please write down the best parts of clinical medicine to help you put things in perspective.

I'm going to give you an assignment. We've thought about what you don't like, and we've thought about what you do. If you could change your practice environment in some reasonable way, would you stay and continue practicing medicine? In other words, is there some form of accommodation that could theoretically be made, and if it were made, you would keep your current job?

Let me give you an example. Let's say you love clinical practice, you love your patients, you love your coworkers, but you just can't stand being on call anymore. If you could get rid of call, but otherwise keep your job similar, would you stay?

Let's say you dream of living in the mountains because you love to ski but you work in Nebraska. Routine skiing is impossible for you. If you could do the same job you're doing now, but skiing was more accessible would you continue practicing clinical medicine? Is there any reasonable accommodation that could be made to help you stay in clinical medicine?

You can often work out a deal with your group or hospital to accommodate your needs because you're a great physician, and they want to keep you. Or you could stay in medicine and work elsewhere still care for patients, and eliminate the irritants driving you up the wall.

Think about that. If you could change call, nights, weekends, holidays, work environment, work location, or even the people you work with, would you be happy? For example, if you're not a big fan of your coworkers but love clinical medicine and don't mind call, you could change groups.

This self-assessment will make a difference as we go forward in this book and decide your best career options. We'll collaborate to determine whether you should stay in medicine or not. How can we make clinical practice work for you? And if we can't, we'll look at alternatives.

If you're sure you want to leave medicine, our next task is to figure out how you want to change your lifestyle in your next career.

You may want something that has fewer total work hours. If you're working 60, 70, or 80 hours a week, you may want a career where you only work 20 or 30 hours. Less work equals more free time for your family and health. Perhaps you want more control over your schedule. Very admirable. I completely understand that. Part of the reason I work per diem and consult with physicians is because it allows me control over my schedule. That means a lot to me.

How about a less stressful job? You may have decided that medicine is too emotionally draining. It's taking too much of a toll on your mental health. There is nothing wrong with feeling that way. I applaud you for being brave and honest enough to say, "Yes, this just isn't working out because this stress or moral injury is more than I would like to have in my life." We can find you a less stressful job.

You might want a job with more travel, either vacation or travel as part of work.

You may want a job that gives you more creativity. As you know, medicine typically doesn't allow for much imagination. If you'd like more creativity in your life, you may need to switch careers or start a creative hobby/side hustle.

Many folks want a job where you can work from home (WFH). I know I do. Fortunately, there are now opportunities within medicine (telemedicine) to WFH while caring for patients. I wanted to be with my kids and family more. It ain't so easy when you're always at work, so at least partial WFH makes sense for my goals.

You want to work from home because you want to live on a boat or move to Europe, Japan, India, or Australia. You obviously can't practice ophthalmology or surgery in The States if you're not physically on site.

Perhaps you feel you're as good as you'll ever be as a doctor and now want a different career. It may not even be an issue of the hours, or the stress, or the location, or the people. You just want to do something else. This makes a lot of sense, and it's not discussed enough. After all, we may be working for 35 or 45 years. Who knows? You might live to be 100 or more.

If you're working for many years to come, you may not want to be doing the same thing that whole time. Frankly, I'm not sure that we are meant to be doing the same career for 50 years. Some people love it. More power to you. A lot of people don't.

You want to start a business or a charity. I'm with you! Creating a new entity from scratch is engaging and creative, opening up new possibilities. Starting a charity allows you to make a difference in the world and help the lives of other people, animals, or whatever it is that you're passionate about. You want time for that.

Perhaps you are someone who went into healthcare, but you always liked research more. You became a doctor because that seemed like the path of least resistance. But there are tons of opportunities in research, which we'll get to a little bit later. That may be your calling, and you should pursue that.

Maybe you want to leave medicine because you want to make more money. I caution you to be careful here. Now, I'm not saying there's anything wrong with wanting to make more money. The trouble is that few fields can pay more money, more reliably than medicine. While investment banking may be an exception, doctors make more money on average than most other professions.

Finally, you may be done with work altogether. Perhaps you want to spend time with your grandkids. You want to spend time with your spouse. You want to travel the world. You aren't physically up to it anymore. You're not mentally up to it anymore. There are many reasons you may decide, "You know what? I'm done with work." And that is alright; just speak to a financial planner first!

Chapter 4

Making Your Clinical Career Work

Do you all remember the Vanilla Ice song? If there's a problem, yo, I'll solve it. Well, he may have been onto something when it comes to salvaging physician clinical careers. I know you're laughing, but bear with me here for a minute. Most physicians I work with aren't looking to leave clinical medicine. Rather, they are dissatisfied with one or more aspects of their job, and they would love to fix it and continue to practice medicine and care for patients. It's only a minority of people who want to leave medicine altogether.

This chapter will focus on how you and I could work together and hopefully find a way to make your clinical career more satisfying where you don't need to leave medicine altogether. For those of you convinced that you want to leave medicine completely, you could skip this chapter, but I would encourage you to read it anyway because I may share some ideas that you haven't considered that might help you stay in clinical medicine and find more joy and meaning in clinical work.

I will mention a few companies, groups, or social media groups in this chapter. I don't have any financial relationship with any of these, and I am not endorsing any of them. I share them as examples. If you decide to follow or speak to any of these companies or groups, please research them before you join.

I hope you took my advice earlier, spent some time on introspection, and thought about what bothers you about your current situation. If you did, that will help you make sensible decisions about what to do going forward. For example, if you figured out that you still love patients or at least like patients enough, and you like your clinical responsibilities, but you have a particular objection, my first tip is to see if you could work with your group or hospital to find a way to solve this.

Let me give examples of some common objections or difficulties people have with work that they could address with their group, which are potentially solvable. Many of these might apply to what's bothering you. These are the big things that bother many of my physician clients. Number one is call. Very few people like call. I certainly did not like call. I can't blame anyone for not wanting to either have to work for 24 or 36 hours in a hospital or have some sort of pager call. It's horrible. I understand that it is needed, and I appreciate people who do call and are putting themselves out there because any one of us, you or I, might need to go into the hospital in the middle of the night as a patient, and I'm thankful someone's there. But from a physician's perspective, call is one of the biggest complaints.

Other common complaints are working on weekends and working nights. Working nights could be either where you literally work overnight or where you have long, unpredictable shifts that run into the nighttime. I would say this is a common one where you think you'll finish around 4:00 or 5:00, but you're there until 8:00. When you're there until 8:00, that may cause you to miss the gym, your family dinner, or your daughter's soccer practice. That kind of stuff wears you down if it happens too often. Another common problem that may be fixable is driving to too many locations. A lot of surgeons work at multiple facilities. For example, I know some pediatric surgeons who work at three or four hospitals. If you live in a busy, big city full of traffic like Los Angeles, it could be very draining for surgeons, anesthesiologists, or other people to drive across the city multiple times per day.

Too many total hours is another common complaint, somewhat different from call or overnights. In other words, perhaps you don't mind working nights, weekends, or holidays. You just don't want to work more than 30 hours a week. If you had the rest of the time free, then you could do the other stuff you want, like time with your spouse, a side project, exercising, playing pickleball, or whatever you like to do. And finally, another common complaint that is fixable within a group is income. Sometimes, people feel that they're not making enough. Perhaps partners are making more than you are. Your compensation from the hospital isn't fair, and you're not happy with your benefits if you are a W-2 employee.

All these issues are potentially solvable if you go and speak to your medical group, especially if you offer to do something in exchange. Your bargaining power will be stronger if they're short-staffed.

Here are some ideas you could offer your group in exchange for concessions elsewhere. These are good food for thought. You'll come up with some of your own ideas. I found a lot of surgeons and OB-GYN doctors who love to do surgery but don't enjoy being in the clinic. If you don't like call, you could work out a deal where you take less call or fewer nights, and in exchange, you would do more clinic time and free your other surgeon or OB-GYN colleagues from clinic. This exchange could be an easy sell in many cases because clinic work is less desirable for many people. Everybody's different.

On a related note, I've also found that many surgeons closing in on retirement don't want to leave clinical medicine altogether. They could no longer work nights or take call. Typically, these senior physicians offer to work in the clinic and allow the other surgeons, the younger surgeons, to spend more time operating, which is what many want to do anyway.

Back to the theme of getting rid of call. You can offer to work extra holidays, work longer days during the daytime, or take longer shifts, for example, rather than take call or work overnight. Alternatively, if you prefer to avoid the unpredictability of call, you could offer to staff a week of nights instead.

A lot of groups have switched to this. Pediatricians, internists, and family medicine doctors use this hospitalist model. Some people don't mind nights. Those people take the nights. You could even pay them more money. It saves the rest of the people from having to take the nights. Other people may want nights because it allows them to be with their kids during the day when their spouse is at work. A lot of nurses do this.

Here are a few other things you might be able to work out in your contract with your existing group. Ask for a sabbatical. Many people like clinical practice. They like what they're doing but want to taste something else. It could be uninterrupted family time. It might be living in another country for six months. It might be researching, experimenting with a startup or charity, or writing a book. It might be working with your child before their bar mitzvah or with your spouse when they train for a marathon. There are a million reasons you might want a prolonged time off.

In my old hospital, Kaiser, they were quite good about this. You were allowed to have a sabbatical after a certain time of service. Typically, you won't get paid for these sabbaticals. You may or may not keep your insurance coverage, but at least it allows you to experience different lifestyles or finish other projects with the comfort of knowing that your job is still waiting for you. And that may be better than quitting altogether.

Here's another idea to offer to your group. Volunteer to take on some of the unsavory administrative tasks. For example, a lot of people don't like doing the schedule. Anesthesiologists or surgeons offer to run the OR board, sit at the desk, and ensure all the rooms run on time and that people go where they're supposed to go. In exchange, you have fewer calls and potentially more predictable days.

If you are in a subspecialty, you constantly seek new patients. For example, if you're a retina surgeon, you need to continually look for new patients, and that often means going out to general ophthalmologists or optometrists and hosting dinners and lunches and this and that as a way of schmoozing these people to send you referrals. The truth is that a lot of doctors don't like doing this. They find it tedious and taxing. Many doctors aren't extroverted and would love to avoid the outreach. If you're extroverted, you could volunteer for these lunches, dinners, and recruiting visits. Then, you share the patients with the group or your hospital. In exchange, you have less call or nights or weekends or whatever.

Finally, another option you can offer your group is to learn a valuable skill so that you can replace paid staff. For example, you could learn about marketing. You could take over some marketing responsibilities the group would otherwise have to farm out. This one is trickier because marketers tend to get paid less than physicians. But you can make the case that, as a doctor, you would be better at marketing medical services than a third-party advertising firm. It's a compelling argument. You should discuss it with your group and see if you can convince them. The same scenario could work for accounting.

All right, you've tried all these things. You spoke to your colleagues; you made all these offers and still could not get the deal you wanted. They said everybody has to take calls, work nights, and work on Thanksgiving or New Year's. If this is unacceptable to you, or you've come to terms with the fact that you don't like your colleagues, there is an easy option - leave and work somewhere else. Do it, and don't feel guilty.

Your problem may be that you don't like where you live. Perhaps you've *never* wanted to live where you are. Or you like where you live but don't like the physical structure of your office/clinic/hospital.

Maybe it's too dark. Perhaps your facility doesn't have the equipment you like, and they'll never get it. Or they won't get the support staff you need, or there's so much administrative work, and you can't see any way out of that because that's just how your group practices, or maybe you aren't a big fan of your patient population for whatever reason. But if you still like patient care, you can solve those problems by changing groups or cities.

I'll tell you about my experience. I worked for a group for a long time. For the first decade, the idea of leaving was almost inconceivable. I was comfortable there. We had an excellent human resources department that took care of me. I was familiar with the hospital and my colleagues. I liked the nurses and support staff. I knew how things worked. So, I stayed.

The path of least resistance is to continue doing the same 'ol, same 'ol even if you are unhappy at work and are not living where you want to live.

It's easy to stay on the treadmill and keep doing what you're doing. Many physicians are conservative in behavior and don't want to rock the boat and do something very different. The easiest thing to do is to stay with the same group. But let me tell you, that isn't how life is outside of medicine.

If you speak to friends in other professions, like lawyers, marketers, investors, or executives, they tend to switch companies every few years. In some ways, that's more common now than it ever was. Outside of medicine, changing locations or companies is expected. It's relatively uncommon in healthcare, but doesn't have to be that way.

If you like what you're doing but don't like where you're doing it, who you're with, or the practice environment, I give you permission to go out and look at working elsewhere. Look at switching cities. Take out a map of the country and open your mind to other places. Look where your brother is living, where your parents are living, or where your childhood best friend is. You may want to move closer to your kids, the beach, the mountains, or the lake. You've been living in a small town and want to try the big city. Or you're tired of the big city and want to try a more rural life. Open your mind to these possibilities. Once you do that, you'll find it's really pretty fun.

I love sitting down in front of my computer. You can open up Google Maps and put a city on the map. There will be a little pin you can hover over to see pictures from that city. How fun is it to go and fantasize about living in all these different places? You can move to a place you know or experiment with one that you don't. The world is yours. If you leave your state and go to another state, you will likely need to get another medical license for the new state. You'll probably need to change your malpractice insurance policy and some other things. Sure, it's a bit of work, but all those tasks are manageable.

Because there is such a shortage of physicians, finding another place to work is easy. If you want to go somewhere else, you have my permission to do it, or you might stay in your city and join a different group (if your contract allows for that). For example, people in Los Angeles might find a better group across town. It's closer to where you live, or you like it more. Give it a shot. Don't be afraid.

All right, the next option I want to share with you is going either per diem or part-time. The way this would work is that you either switch groups and do it with a group that would allow you to or stay with your group and do it. Many groups won't give you all these concessions about call, but they will, interestingly enough, often let you work per diem or part-time. The reason they'll give you all these goodies if you work per diem or part-time is you'll save them money on benefits, and they might like the fact that they could potentially plug you in on days that they're short and not have you sit around on days where they're overstaffed.

Let me give you an example. Say you want more time off work to do other things and don't mind working weekends and holidays. You could work per diem or part-time and fill in on the weekends, on the holidays, on that Wednesday when three people want off for their birthdays at the same time, for spring break when people are going out with their families on vacation. When you do that, your groups will love you because they're happy to have you take those days they don't want.

And many groups are happy with it because they're not obligating themselves to you. In other words, they only use you as much as they want, not more than that.

The downside to this strategy is that the groups may not need you next month or next year. So, to do this, you need to have a risk tolerance and money in the bank so that if you don't get as many shifts or days as you expect, you're still okay and won't get kicked out of your house.

When I left my long-term hospital job, this is what I did. I started working per diem in many different groups, and the reason I worked for multiple groups was that I wanted to see what these other groups were like. I worked for one system for a long time. I didn't know what else was out there. So, for me, it was fun. I'm an anesthesiologist. I did dental cases with a dental anesthesia group and had a great time. They flew me around to different dental offices across the state of California. I would go in, do cases for a few days, and fly back. They put me in hotels. I had a good time, and it was fun doing something different.

I was also able to do dental cases in my own town. I didn't always have to fly, but flying was part of the fun for me. On top of that, I did per diem work in Beverly Hills in plastic surgeons' offices, and that was a fun opportunity for me to work with some of the world's top plastic surgeons. I saw how influencers, people you and I see all the time on Instagram or TikTok, look the way they do. Trust me, folks, it isn't all natural. I enjoyed that. What was good about it was that I worked the days I wanted to work, and I didn't work the days I didn't. I only worked as much as I wanted to work. If my kids were starting school, a family member needed me, or I wanted to do something on a random Thursday or a particular weekend, I didn't work then because I had control of my schedule.

I didn't have call. I didn't work on the weekends with this arrangement or nights, and it was fun. But, I did work with several different groups. I did that partly because I was worried that if one group decided they didn't need me anymore, didn't like me, or their business dried up, or only wanted me for days I couldn't work, I would have options.

I worked for several groups because I wanted the ability to walk away from something that I didn't like. This doesn't happen often, but occasionally, you don't like a facility. This rarely happened to me, but it did happen once.

As part of one of my PRN groups where I worked, we would go to a nearby surgery center. Initially, I liked the place. We were doing the types of cases that I enjoyed, and the days were reasonable in length, and I thought the surgeons were competent. It was a good environment. But then, they changed the center's manager. They hired a new administrator with no experience - the former social media manager!

This person had no clue how to run a surgery center. They had no training, no experience, and no qualifications. They were friends with the owner. That's how they got the job. Naturally, this person was not able to retain staff. They looked at the staff in the center as warm bodies to fill a chair rather than as a team. In a relatively short time, all, and I mean all the experienced nurses left. All the experienced scrub techs left. Even the front desk staff who checked in patients suffered high turnover.

Eventually, all the support staff, from the nurses to the scrub techs, were agency people or per diems. And I kid you not when I say there was a day I went there when every single person was a per diem, and the most experienced person at the center was a per diem who was there the day before. In other words, the senior people had one day of onsite experience. Anyone who knows about the benefits of teams in medicine knows this is a disaster. So, I left. It was too unsafe.

I tell you that story not because it is common but because it is rare. Most importantly, I tell you that story because I had my finger in several pots. I was doing per diem in several places. As soon as I felt this place was unsafe, I could walk away without worrying. I didn't need to stay in something that I did not like. That's per diem. I'm a big fan, and I recommend it to many of the physicians I work with. I would love to talk to you more about it.

My story notwithstanding, per diem is a fantastic opportunity to work in different places, enjoy some variety, work as much or as little as you wish, leave environments you don't like, and stay in places you do.

Part-time is a little different than per diem. Part-time typically means you agree to work for your group, but you work 60% or 80% instead of being a full-time person. I did this for several years at my old hospital before I left. I worked 80% for a while and then switched to 60%. There are a million different ways to structure part-time arrangements. It could be that an 80% person does precisely the same stuff that everybody does, but only 80% of it. So you take 80% of the call, 80% of the weekends, and 80% of the holidays you would have taken. Or other groups might try to extract a pound of flesh and say, "Well, you can work 80% of the days, but you still have to take the same call as everybody else." Some places will say, "If you're part-time, you can keep all your benefits, like your health insurance." Other sites may say, "If you don't work a certain amount, you lose your benefits." There are different deals you could work out.

Part-time is an excellent option for many people. As I said, I did it myself for a couple of years before I left entirely to become a per diem. It's comfortable; you know the people you're with; you're still working in the same environment you already know; you might be able to keep your benefits. I was able to do that. And you don't have as much call or as many nights as you had when you were working full-time. You'll make less money, but you need to accept that trade-off.

There is another option I have yet to see, but I'm advocating to anyone who will listen to me. I mentioned this in online discussion forums with executives and directly with physicians in the trenches. My idea is a variant of 80% time. Google had something like this for their engineers. The way Google did it was they said that you have to spend 80% of your time working on stuff you needed to do for your job, whatever your job assignments were. But for 20% of their time, they could work on their own project that somehow related to Google, but it was a project of their choice.

People love this because it allows them to be creative. If your thing is that you like your job, you like what you're doing, you enjoy your colleagues, you like your patients, but you wish you had some more time for some creative outlet, this could be the answer for you.

If you're a hospital administrator, please consider offering this option or contact me to discuss it. Many of the coolest things that came out of Google happened because they had smart, talented people who were allowed to let their minds wander, and they came up with ways of helping the system independently. From what I understand, Gmail came out of this and some other neat stuff.

If a doctor could get 20% time to explore creative projects, he or she could develop new clinical pathways, improve efficiency, or find new ways to administer the medical group. They may go through and look at the equipment in the hospital and say, "Hey, this stuff is garbage. Let's get rid of it and replace it with something else."

There are a million things that an intelligent person, with some free time and creative energy, could produce. I hope more people will consider this; it's not common now. But working part-time, where you make 80% or 60% of your salary, does exist. I recommend taking that up if you're looking for a change but are not quite ready to leave. I did it. I was happy with it for a few years until I didn't want to be on call anymore, and I didn't want to work at night anymore. Even with 60% or 80% of the call and night responsibility, I couldn't do it.

Switching gears, you can preserve your clinical practice but make life easier or different by practicing more telemedicine. I will toot my own horn and say I was into this several years ago. Telemedicine is uncommon for anesthesiologists. But years ago, I had the idea of setting up my consultation practice where I would help athletes with nutrition and general health and wellness. And there are several platforms where a doctor could hang up their online shingle. You need some form of advertising to draw people to you. Then, you could provide medical consultation and get paid for telemedicine.

This type of telemedicine has some pluses and minuses. The pluses are that you are your own boss, you work as much or as little as you want to, and you can focus on things that interest you. The minuses are that you must be careful that your malpractice insurance covers what you're discussing. This was a challenge for me because, as an anesthesiologist, some malpractice carriers would say, "Well, who are you to talk about nutrition? You can't recommend eating broccoli." I know that sounds crazy, but that is actually what some carriers said. And, of course, the other downside is you have to do some old-fashioned marketing. You have to bring patients to you, which might appeal to some of you and turn others off. Again, if you're interested in this, talk to me. I could tell you how to do it.

But there are other more established ways to do telemedicine where you could work for your group or your hospital. And there are now medical practices that focus on telemedicine or have telemedicine mixed in with the in-person stuff. Telemedicine is a natural fit for certain specialties. Suppose you're an internist, a pediatrician, or a family medicine doctor. In that case, you can see a good percentage of patients using telemedicine. Then, you direct the other patients who cannot be seen remotely to an in-person clinic or emergency room. Whether you're an emergency medicine or an ICU doctor, telemedicine urgent care is phenomenal. If you're in certain types of surgery, like a general surgeon or even a plastic surgeon for pre- and post-op visits, or if you're an OB-GYN and want to see patients remotely for part of your practice, you can do that.

With telemedicine, you typically enjoy more control over your hours. You can work from home. A lot of people who are physician parents, for example, want to keep practicing, but they really want to be there to get their kids ready for the school bus. If you're doing telemedicine all or part of the time, you could be home, prepare your kids for the school bus, and then hop on your telemedicine calls.

Telemedicine is growing in fields that you may not expect. Dermatology can lend itself to telemedicine. A lot of eye doctors can potentially work through telemedicine, as crazy as it sounds.

I want to tell you a story. I knew someone who needed to go and get new glasses. They went into the optometrist's office, and the optometrist wasn't physically there!

The onsite optician did a few measurements, and then the optometrist appeared on a view screen. The optometrist could adjust the lenses that the patient was looking through remotely. They even took a picture of the retina and sent it to the optometrist. Again, this technology is evolving. It will be used more.

Another exciting use of telemedicine is dental. There's even teledentistry, where someone goes to the office and gets their teeth cleaned by the dental assistant, and the dentist is not physically there. I have doubts about this one because I'd rather my dentist actually touch my teeth, but I know this can work. We will see this innovation throughout the medical world.

Locum tenens. I love this topic, and many physicians I speak with are curious about it. I want to demystify it for you, tell you what it is, what's great about it, what are some risks with it, and help nudge you in this direction because I'm a big fan.

When I left my hospital job, I worked per diem for several years and mixed in some locums. I went to a children's hospital that I liked in Central California. It was a great place; the facility was fantastic; the people were wonderful; the medical care there was excellent; the work hours were acceptable, and the patients were great. There were lots of needy kids and appreciative families.

They had trouble recruiting people to move there permanently because it was in the middle of the state, and not many doctors wanted to move to that city. I would travel there for a week, and the locums company would either pay for me to drive or they would fly me there. They put me in a hotel and gave me a rental car if I flew there. I would work for my shift, and then I would explore the town, hang out in the hotel, and recharge before the next day. I did this for a week at a time and would do it here or there when I wanted to.

For me, it worked out well. I wasn't ready to give up hospital practice entirely, and all the PRN stuff I was doing was in clinics. It allowed me to maintain my tertiary practice. It worked out because it was a reliable, high-paying job. I love to travel, so it was fun because I got to stay in a hotel, see a different city, and practice in a wonderful place.

What I did wouldn't work for everyone and wouldn't have worked for me long-term because, eventually, I would not have wanted to be away from my family for a week at a time. I've known other physicians who have done this long-term. For some people, it works out great even with their family because they travel for locum tenens for a week or maybe for two weeks a month, and then the rest of the time, they are with their spouse and their kids. For them, it works out because they'd rather have this period of concentrated work and then no work at all versus the standard model where you're working continuously.

These docs doing long-term locum tenes enjoyed control over their schedule because they decided which weeks they worked. If their family wanted to take a vacation for two or three weeks, they could. It may work well for other people who don't have kids or those who can take their family with them.

A quick aside. One time, I took a traveling per diem dental anesthesia assignment. I took the whole family with me to another town in California. We stayed in an Airbnb with a pool. Everybody had a blast, and the Airbnb was free, and I was paid to be there! The kids loved it, and so did my parents. We still love to reminisce about that trip.

What are locums? Locum tenens is when a hospital, surgery center, urgent care, or any practice setting that employs physicians needs physicians to come part-time or here or there. They might have a few one-off understaffed days. Perhaps they need someone on October 31st because everybody's out for Halloween. They could need someone for four months because somebody is on maternity leave. They may need extra people to hold them over until they hire someone else, either because someone is leaving or business is increasing. So they depend on locums to fill in the gaps, but whatever the arrangement is, they're all more or less similar, and here's how it works.

You can find ads for these locum positions on your specialty's job websites, employment forums like Indeed, or the locum companies themselves. I tell you, once the locum companies know that you're in the market, they will message you every other day with opportunities. I am constantly getting text messages, calls, and emails from these locums companies saying they have an opportunity here or there. Since I'm licensed in three states, I constantly get tons of unsolicited opportunities to work. Some of the bigger locum companies are CompHealth or Staff Care, but there are many.

Locum companies are like recruiters. They run ads. They reach out to their network, whatever they do, and they try to find physicians like you or me to come in and fill the spot. They know a lot about the position they're looking to fill. They will know whether it involves call, nights, or weekends. They should know the approximate hours required. For example, "This job is from 7:00 AM to 3:00 PM Monday through Friday." They'll know how many days you have to work.

They'll say, "You have to work October 2nd and 15th. If you want this, it's just those two days." Or they may say, "We have an ongoing need for months; take as many days as you want." Or they may say, "They're looking for people to work a week at a time. Can you commit to doing that?" Or they might say, "It's ongoing. We're looking for people to work at least three days a week for the next few months. Can you do that?" All kinds of different arrangements. They'll be able to tell you about the practice environment, like, are you working solo or with others? Are you supervising mid-level providers or not? And they'll, of course, know the city.

Locums usually include malpractice insurance, including a tail for whatever work you do with them. So if you work a couple of days here or there, you work a week, a month, whatever it is, typically locums companies will provide you with malpractice insurance with a tail for this.

This benefit is especially valuable if you let your malpractice insurance lapse. Or you're closing in on retirement but want to do some extra shifts but don't want to keep malpractice policies, or if you're licensed in multiple states, you may not have malpractice insurance in all the states. There are a lot of benefits to having the locums company provide the malpractice. One cool thing you could do is build a practice that is entirely locums. You can get by without a malpractice policy and use the policies they give you. You save a bundle that way, and I admire people who can do that.

The way locum companies typically pay is much easier than any other medical job. Most locum arrangements will pay you by the hour worked, and they pay you every week or every two like clockwork. It's easy. It's deposited directly into your account. What's nice about this is that it doesn't involve any insurance billing, and you are not involved in billing the medical group or anything like that. There's no getting your hands dirty with the money. I'm speaking in general. Of course, some companies may be exceptions, so you have to do your own research.

But the typical way it would work is they will say, for example, "We will pay you X dollars per hour with an eight-hour minimum per day." So, if you work five days this week, you'll get paid for eight hours a day at the agreed-upon rate, even if you only work four or six hours. If you work more than eight hours, they typically have an overtime rate that is agreed on in advance. Most places don't want you working overtime because it costs them too much, but sometimes you will, and it's all paid out.

If the patient's insurance carrier refuses to pay, it doesn't matter. If the medical group takes a while paying, it doesn't matter. The locums company pays you. Again, do your own research, but typically, you will get paid regardless of what happens.

Let me give you an example. Let's say you are an anesthesiologist and are supposed to work at a facility for eight hours at an agreed-upon hourly rate. You're there, but no patient comes in for the first four hours. You're just sitting there reading a book, staring out the window, and thinking how lucky you are to have this job. The next hour, you do an appendectomy on a patient without insurance. And then after that, the hospital says, look, we don't need you anymore, and you leave.

You were supposed to be there for eight hours. You were only there for five or six hours. You only worked for one hour in the OR, and that one hour was for an uninsured patient. In some practice environments, on a day like that, you might go home and make $0 if you depend on insurance billing. If you're paid by the hour by the hospital, you might be paid for just the hours you were there. But if you did that as a locum, you would've been paid for the whole eight-hour day even though you didn't make the hospital or the medical group any money. I want to say that again. You would've been paid for your agreed-upon rate for the whole day even though you did not make any money for the hospital or medical group. You are not worried about that. Your only worry is being there on time, providing excellent medical care (as you always should), and then going home when your shift is over. In exchange for that, you get paid a guaranteed amount.

Another key feature of locums is the travel. Some locum opportunities are very close to you. They may be just across town or, if lucky, even closer than your current job. You drive to them, and that's great. Others may be further away across the state, for example, like what I did. Depending on your lifestyle, this may be a plus or minus. But here's what can make locums either great or horrible for you. You can travel far distances with locums if you wish to.

Let's say, like me, you're licensed in multiple states. I'm licensed in California, Texas, and Georgia. I live in Georgia now, but I used to live in California and Texas. For my lifestyle, I want to stay in Georgia at this point, but I constantly get messages for opportunities in California or Texas. I could take some of those opportunities in other states or even across Georgia. I could go to Savannah, which is a beautiful city. I could go. I could work, and I could travel and see other places. And I could have fun being in different areas and then return home. The company covers all that travel, the hotel, the plane, and everything.

I don't want to do that at this point in my life because I don't want to be away from my kids that long, but I have done that, and maybe in the future, I would like to do that, but certainly, some people love the experience. Either it works better with their childcare arrangements, they don't have kids, or they take their kids with them.

Another neat thing is that you could work with locum companies and go to places where you do not have a license. For example, some areas typically have lots of need, like Alaska. There may be needs in exotic locations like Hawaii or Maine, and the locums companies, in many situations, especially if you agree to go for a certain amount of time, will even license you in these other states. For example, in my case, say there's a need in a city in Montana. Perhaps I've always wanted to go to Montana to see what it's like to be out there, in the fields and open skies. I'm not licensed there, and doing that wouldn't be worth my trouble.

But a locums company may say, "Well, if you agree to go there for this assignment one week a month for the next five months," or whatever they need, they will license you there. They will fill out the application and pay the application fee. Of course, they'll need to ask you some questions because they won't know the answer to everything, but they do all the hard work, arrange the licensing, and, as I mentioned, the malpractice insurance. What a great way to collect medical licenses in multiple states for free!

There are some disadvantages of locums that you should know about. Tomorrow is not guaranteed. There may be tons of opportunities now. But those opportunities may not be there in three months. That could be because they have fewer patients, hired someone, or don't like working with you. You have to have a risk tolerance for this. The risk is lower the more flexible you are about where you're willing to travel or if you take multiple assignments. But there is some risk, and you must be comfortable with that.

As an aside, remaining in your regular job has risks. Nothing is risk-free. Your current employer may decide to switch groups, or they may not have enough patients to keep all the staff. Your hospital may even close. Nothing is risk-free, but working locums is a greater risk for most people than staying in their current jobs.

Another disadvantage of locums is that they typically don't have any benefits other than the malpractice insurance I mentioned earlier. Most assignments will not include health, life, or disability insurance. If that's important to you, you'll need to figure out how to get that on your own. This is also true with per diem type work, where none of those would typically be included.

You don't get paid days off. If you have a W-2 job, you would typically enjoy some paid holidays. You might have some paid sick leave. Locums and per diem usually do not have that benefit, so if you take a day off or are ill and can't go to work, you don't make any money that day.

You're generally paid as a 1099 employee. There may be some exceptions to this by company and state, but that's the usual arrangement. I'm not a tax advisor, so I cannot give you any tax advice. I recommend that you speak to your accountant. When you're paid as a 1099 employee, there are some tax implications, potentially good or bad. You should understand what they are, particularly if you are used to a W-2 job.

In summary, I'm a big advocate of locums. Some relatively large, well-established companies are reasonably trustworthy, although you should do your own research. These companies allow you to work in various practice settings near and far. They can help you find other jobs in your state or other states. They can help you get licensed in other states. They pay you promptly, and typically, it's not dependent on insurance or billing. They pay easily and frequently. If you don't like the assignment, you can leave once it's over. It can be fun to go to other places. Best of all, you have control over your schedule. If an assignment isn't when you want or where you want, doesn't pay you enough, or doesn't appeal to you for whatever reason, you don't take it. No problem.

The disadvantage is that these assignments could end at any time, so there's some risk that you won't get long-term employment. They typically don't provide benefits other than malpractice and travel. And for some people, it may be a disadvantage to be paid with a 1099. You'll have to speak to your tax planner.

Let's talk about research. This is one that I don't have much personal experience with. I haven't had much interest in doing research. But I do want to give a few perspectives about this to give you some ideas about research that you can keep in mind if this appeals to you. When we work together, I would happily review these options with you. We could research how to do research, but here are a couple of things I'd like you to consider if research appeals to you.

Number one, depending on your practice setting, you might be able to incorporate research into your clinical practice. For example, if you're working at an academic hospital, a VA, or even some larger private practice groups, there may be ways that you could do research in addition to clinical. In other words, you'd split your time. For those who like clinical medicine but want to do it less, doing some research is an excellent opportunity to keep the clinical exposure but have a little more variety.

Alternatively, although it's not the subject of this chapter, you could consider leaving clinical medicine altogether and only doing research. Whether you continue to do clinical medicine along with research depends on your taste and where you're working. Some facilities, like an academic hospital, will probably expect that you still do some clinical practice. In contrast, if you left and did research for a pharmaceutical company, you may be unable to do clinical practice even if you wanted to.

There are several different types of research. Of course, there's clinical research where you investigate how medications, protocols, or other treatment plans impact patient outcomes. There's pharmaceutical research, where you look more at drug development or trials. There's basic science research where you're working in the lab. There's nonclinical research where you look at hospital efficiency or ways to improve patient satisfaction. Does adding more light or plants to rooms improve patient satisfaction, length of stay, etc?

I mentioned this because some people love bench research. You may like the idea of research but not bench research. You might want to do some of this nonclinical stuff working for pharmaceutical companies or develop patient treatment plans in hospitals or medical centers. All these are options, and you should find out which, if any, of these appeal to you.

There are tons of places you can work and do research. Academic hospitals and the VA spring to mind. You could join a pharmaceutical company and be a research coordinator there. If you're in a private group, you could do some nonclinical research. Another option is to join a startup or a small company looking for an expert research consultant.

In other words, your pharmaceutical research doesn't necessarily need to be at a large pharma company. It could be at a startup with its advantages of potentially being more fun and faster-paced, and you might get paid with stock options. But the usual startup disadvantages are there, like lower base salary, greater unpredictability, that type of thing. Research is a great option to add to or replace your clinical job.

Hospital leadership. This is something that I have done, and I enjoyed it. I was the head of my pediatric anesthesia group at our medical center for many years. That responsibility gave me some fun things to do, like making the schedule and improving OR utilization. I did some teaching. I frequently worked with the radiology department because we would coordinate new ways of delivering sedated MRIs and CT scans. I worked with the surgery department, pediatricians, and hospital administration. I enjoyed it because it allowed me to support the medical center while not being 100% clinical. It was a fun variety for me, and I liked it. It didn't save me from call or overnight shifts, but at least some days were broken up, and I was doing something different than simply being in the operating room the whole day.

Hospital leadership could also involve teaching. You can teach residents, fellows, mid-level providers, nurses, medical students, or college students. You could be part of the upper-level hospital leadership where you are the medical director, the CEO, or you're on committees within the hospital. There are a million ways of arranging hospital leadership, and some facilities even require that you do at least some leadership, research, or teaching. Every place is different.

Hospital leadership is ideal for people who still want to practice clinical medicine but want more variety or control over their practice environment or creative output. It may be something for you if you like going to meetings like interfacing with people from other departments. Hospital leadership can replace a clinical career if you prefer. There are some situations where the higher-up physician administrators of the hospital do that full-time and don't do any clinical care anymore. And there are other environments where the head physician administrators of the hospital still do clinical care. Each place, again, is different.

There's a massive demand for physician leaders, and the hospital where you work now may need them. Or if not, plenty of other places would hire you if you want to do that. Some might expect you to have an advanced degree, like an MBA or a master's in public health; others don't. Many would be happy to have you in hospital leadership if you have relevant experience. For example, if you were the head of your subgroup like I was, or if you've served on some hospital committees, that may be sufficient in the eyes of the hiring managers to put you in a hospital leadership position.

If you're interested in doing this, there are several ways you could research it, and one of the ways is through networking forums. There's a place on LinkedIn, the Physician Leadership Networking Forum, which has many opportunities. Or check out another company, PracticeMatch. Again, I don't have any financial relationship with them and don't endorse them, but those are two options that you could look into, or there are many others. You can go to Indeed or Glassdoor and find hospital leadership opportunities.

The next thing is medical philanthropy. I'm distinguishing medical philanthropy from other philanthropic projects that are nonclinical. For this chapter, I want to focus on clinical charitable projects. Again, there are several different ways you could do this.

Back where I used to work at Kaiser, we had many people who volunteered to help others internationally. Kaiser, to their credit, was very supportive. They would take a week or two off and fly to other countries like Guatemala to help with medical missions. They would care for underserved communities that needed surgery, anesthesia, or primary care. I haven't personally done this, but I knew many people who did, and I've spoken to them at great length. If you're interested, medical missions are a fun and satisfying way to aid needy people.

It's also a great way to keep your clinical skills up if you're nearly retired but still looking to do some clinical work. Many physicians who have just retired from their regular practice will do these medical missions for a year or a couple of years, off and on, to give back to the community and maintain their clinical skills. Several organizations could help you do this if you need help knowing where to begin. Again, I don't endorse any of these, but some include Doctors Without Borders, which can go into several different situations to help people in need.

The International Medical Corps or Mercy Ships are another option. You work on floating hospitals. So cool! Their website said that around 50% of the world's population lives near a coast. When the ship goes out and docks at a port, it can access many underserved people. As I understand it, most of their work is in Sub-Saharan Africa. Their website says many of these regions have only two physicians per 10,000 people, so many suffer and die from treatable illnesses. If life on a boat helping underserved communities appeals to you, I would encourage you to research and check that out. They have some pictures on the website showing the cabin and the kids and adults you could help with. And I'm sure you would develop lifelong friends and memories by doing something like that.

Another option to change up your clinical career is to move and practice internationally. I was recently in Europe. We went to the United Kingdom and France and had a fantastic time. I'm embarrassed to say I haven't been to the UK before. We just went on vacation and were there for a few weeks. The people were kind. There were so many beautiful, breathtaking sites to see. We took the kids with us, and they loved it. Truth be told, the kids didn't want to come back. They were having such a good time seeing another country.

It is entirely doable if you want to work internationally as a physician. I started researching this because I wanted to see whether it would make sense for us to go internationally for a year and give the kids an opportunity to live abroad, allow myself to live overseas, and see what medical systems were like elsewhere. If we work together, we can go into this in more detail, but there are ways to do it. Some countries are much easier to go to than others. You have to worry about medical licensing in other countries. Some places make getting a medical license easy if you're already licensed in the US. Other nations make it a big production.

In addition, you have to consider all the usual stuff of moving to another country, like how to pay your taxes. Where do you find a place to live? How do you get health insurance? What are you going to do with your kid's school? What do you do with the house in The States you live in now? There's a lot to consider. But if you're interested in doing it, there are people who will help.

There's a Facebook group that's quite popular called Hippocratic Adventures that you might want to ask to join, and you can connect with many people who have done this. There are also international locum firms like Global Medical Staffing that you might want to research. If you're willing to be flexible about where you go, this is well within your reach if you're interested in it.

This would be a lot of fun, and I'm still considering it. Although, at this point, the logistics of it may be too complex for me in my current situation. But I'd be happy to help support you, and I encourage you to think about it if you'd like to see what it's like to live in another country. You may have relatives in another country and want to live near them. You may wish to sample another country before ultimately moving there. There are a lot of good reasons to go. You'll benefit both as a person and as a clinician. It is possible. But know that there are quite a few logistical hurdles you have to overcome.

The final thing I would like to discuss about changing your clinical career is something I don't recommend, although people talk about it often, and that's changing medical specialties. For example, you're a surgeon, don't like surgery anymore, and are considering a psychiatry residency. Or you're a pediatrician wanting to become an orthopedic surgeon. If this is your dream, and you've thought a lot about it and know what you're doing, go for it. I don't want to be the person to cast out on your dreams. I support you if you want to do it. But unless you are sure this is what you want to do, I would discourage this.

Here's why. To change careers within medicine, you have the same runway problem we discussed earlier. You have to go back to residency and potentially fellowship. You'll go through many years of hard work and call. You won't be paid well. You'll have to do what other people above you tell you to do, which is something you may not be used to because you may not have had to do that for a while. You must match into a residency program, which may not be where you want to live. And then after doing all that, you may end up having to move somewhere you don't want to live to get a job in your new field, or the job you thought you could get isn't there anymore, or you might do all that and then realize that you don't like the new field, or worst of all, you might do all that and realize the problem wasn't the field you're in now. You just don't like clinical medicine, period. You wasted all that time doing a new residency, only to discover that you don't want to do clinical medicine.

Unless you're 100% sure, don't change specialties.

There are things you could do short of that. For example, if you're an emergency medicine doctor and don't like working in the ER, say because of the stress or the overnight hours, you could switch and work in urgent care. Or if you're an internist who doesn't like outpatient stuff, you might become a hospitalist. Or, if you're a hospitalist tired of the inpatient stuff, you can try outpatient telemedicine. Or, if you are a pediatric rheumatologist, for example, and you don't like rheumatology, you could become a general pediatrician. Some of these may require a little training, but it's much easier than it would be if you switched careers within medicine altogether. I recommend doing one of those rather than swapping specialties.

This is the perfect segue to the next chapter, where we'll look at nonclinical careers that might appeal to you as a physician.

Chapter 5

Careers Beyond Medicine

All right, so you've tried everything. You tried to get rid of call, you tried not to work nights. Maybe you worked out a deal where you didn't work on holidays. Perhaps you've tried switching groups or moving to a different city. You've done everything you could. And no matter what, you simply don't like medicine anymore. You gave it your best shot, and you're just not that into clinical medicine.

And that's okay. Not everybody is. Maybe you never were meant to go into it in the first place, and perhaps you were railroaded into medical school by family or friends. Or people change. Maybe you liked it once and don't like it anymore. It can be frustrating, emotionally taxing, draining. It's not for everybody and not for everybody for their whole lives. I get it. I understand that.

I was pushing you to consider clinical careers or alternatives first because I believe in the importance of medicine and taking care of patients. And we need doctors. We need doctors, but it's not for everybody. And the last thing I want you to do is to be unhappy with your work. And that's why I'm here to work with you now to find alternative careers.

You might love medicine but be unable to do it anymore. For example, maybe you're not physically able to do it because of some handicap or chronic medical condition. Perhaps you've lost your license because you let it lapse for too long, or you had substance or malpractice issues that prevented you from maintaining your license.

Or maybe you've retired from a long, satisfying clinical career and want to do something else. You want to use your talents but don't want to return to medicine. Returning to the office or the operating room doesn't appeal to you. This chapter is for you.

I will list some of the more common nonclinical careers I advocate clinicians enter if they want to quit medicine altogether.

You can, if you wish, do some of the following jobs while maintaining a clinical career. You can do some of these part-time. So, I would encourage you to read this chapter, even if you've decided to keep practicing medicine, because some of these might be great side gigs or things you want to do when you eventually retire. After all, that day will likely come at some point. This list isn't in any particular order, but go through it, listen to the different options, and see which of these appeal to you. And then let's talk.

The first one is something in finance or more hardcore business. That would include venture capital, investment banking, or private equity. I want to briefly describe what these are.

The basic idea is that venture capital (VC) firms invest in middle or late-stage startups or smaller established companies. By bringing in money, investment, and expertise, these smaller companies hope to grow, become much more successful, and eventually sold. So, VC firms give other companies operating capital, advice, and then try to sell them later.

Private equity (PR) firms are somewhat similar. They often purchase distressed companies that are not doing well or buy promising early companies. The PE firms give these companies money and expertise, try to revamp or shape them up, and then sell them later. Private equity has become a hot topic in healthcare because many private equity firms are buying physician practices. Private equity firms bought the anesthesia and GI groups in several cities where I've lived.

These medical groups were happy to sell themselves to private equity companies because they were paid handsomely for the sale. The private equity companies often did the administrative work these groups did not want to do. The docs in the group wanted to focus on practicing medicine.

Some doctors enjoyed being part of the PE firm's umbrella. Other doctors working for these private equity-purchased firms were unhappy because they had a new boss, who was typically not a physician. I won't get into the benefits or disadvantages of it, but you should understand that this is happening.

And then a third option would be investment banking. Investment banking is a high-powered business field that typically requires an MBA and a lot of hard work. They help companies buy other companies, merge with other companies, that type of thing.

If any of these finance fields appeal to you, they have some real benefits. They can be very, very interesting and would give your brain an opportunity to do something vastly different than your physician day job.

You could be in demand at these firms, especially those with a healthcare focus. These firms may be happy to have a clinician, especially if you have some business experience, join them as an employee or consultant. They want your expertise. If they're looking at buying or fixing up a health organization, they may be happy to have a doctor on their team who understands the market.

These jobs are appealing because they typically pay well. As I mentioned earlier in the book, there are very few jobs that, on average, pay more than medicine. But finance jobs, especially if you're successful, can be more lucrative than medicine. This is one of the outliers. So, if your goal is to increase your income, although this isn't risk-free, these jobs should be on your radar.

There are some disadvantages to finance jobs. They're highly competitive. There aren't millions of these positions; you must devote time to networking. Many of these positions may require either business experience or an MBA. If this is an avenue you want to take, you could consider getting an MBA or working on an executive MBA part-time while you're still working. These jobs are typically very time-consuming. If you're leaving medicine because you thought medicine was too much work, these jobs may not suit you.

On the other hand, if you're leaving medicine because you don't like patients or just don't like being a doctor but don't mind the work, these jobs may be excellent opportunities - if you don't mind the networking.

The next category of jobs is the pharmaceutical industry. Drug companies love having physicians work for them, especially if you are a physician who works in a particularly lucrative field for the industry.

Oncology springs to mind, or cardiology. Those specialties utilize expensive medications.

Any physician can potentially work for the pharmaceutical industry. If you want to do this, the benefits are that there are lots of different types of jobs within pharma that you could do. For example, you could work in the marketing department. I actually did this when I was in medical school. I worked for the marketing department of a large pharmaceutical company for a couple of months during two summers. It was a great experience. I saw how pharmaceutical companies create outreach plans for physicians to get them to use their products. It was fascinating.

What the pharmaceutical companies do and how they reach out to physicians significantly impact clinical practice. It's intriguing to peek behind the curtain. And it was fun working there. The office was sharp, the people there were bright, and we had access to a lot of data and technology. I thought it was a great experience.

You could also work in drug development. If you're more interested in the research side, you could work for a pharmaceutical company in the lab.

There may even be opportunities to be an executive, particularly if you don't mind working your way up and have some business experience. Again, business experience is helpful here. An MBA is beneficial but not necessary.

As an aside, I had a call the other day from a physician who lost his license some years ago due to substance abuse issues. He wanted to work but could not work in a clinical career. Pharma is an excellent option for someone in that situation.

You might want to consider being a pharmaceutical sales rep or a drug rep. You know, the folks who meet with doctors and try to get them to use their products.

Your initial instinct here might be that this isn't something a doctor should do, or perhaps it's beneath you. I disagree. I know a lot of drug and device reps. They're brilliant people, capable people with great energy and enthusiasm. They have an impact because they go out and educate doctors about new products. Also, these reps are paid quite well. They often get a company car. There are a lot of perks.

So if you've let your license lapse, or if you simply want to go out and about, if you like socializing, and you're not trying to do big strategic projects, being a pharmaceutical rep is definitely an option.

The next option is teaching. I'd like to open your eyes to the wide variety of teaching possibilities. You and I are used to teaching residents, fellows, or medical students. There are many teaching options, even if you don't have a license.

There's teaching within the medical industry itself. And that could be, for example, teaching at an advanced practice nursing school. You could, for example, teach CRNAs or nurse practitioners in training. They need good people.

You can teach medical students and residents, even if you're not working clinically in their specific field of study.

You could teach the pharmaceutical reps because they need to understand the medical concepts related to the drugs or devices they're selling. They would be delighted to have you as a teacher.

You could also teach outside of medicine altogether in colleges. There are a lot of college courses that you could lead, including at business schools, by the way. Business schools want to better understand the health system. They would love to have someone who was a frontline health worker like you. Or you could teach in advanced degree programs like a master's in public health. You could teach health policy or get an MPH yourself.

And finally, I would like you to consider teaching lower grades, like high school, middle school, and elementary school. I suggested teaching younger grades to the physician I mentioned earlier, the one who lost his license due to substance issues. As a society, we need more talented teachers like you throughout the grade spectrum.

Think about it. Plus, you get the perk of having summers off. You feel good that you're helping the community. You get a lot of the emotional benefits of being a physician because you're helping others, you're helping young minds, and you don't have a lot of the same stresses.

Another career to consider is consulting. In this case, you would typically provide your medical expertise to companies in need. There are a few different ways you could go into consulting. You could either join one of the large consulting firms where you are, in a sense, their employee, and they will farm you out to different projects. Or, you can consult directly without the intermediary.

For example, you might work for a consulting firm, and then the consulting firm might send you to a project at, let's say, an underperforming hospital that's losing money and needs to revamp its operations. Or you might be sent to an insurance company or a government office that needs to change their healthcare operations. You're creatively deploying your medical experience.

Alternatively, you can consult for startups.

I do this. There's a startup I consult with that makes respiratory devices. As an anesthesiologist, I have good insight into breathing and can bring much to the table.

When you do these jobs, you typically would be available to answer questions. Maybe the CEO or someone in the company needs some guidance about a medical issue, or they might have questions about what might appeal to doctors or patients. As the consultant, you make yourself available from time to time if they have these questions.

It would be rare for you to be able to do this full-time. Or if you did, it would be temporary because, usually, these companies already have a product close to completion. They want to figure out, for example, if doctors prefer this or that feature. Or would there be any value in putting this extra feature into the product, or is that a waste of time? Those are the kinds of questions they'll ask you.

Consulting, again, is fun. It's creative. You could be making a big difference if you're part of a product that then gets launched. But it does have the disadvantage of not being a reliable source of significant income over the long term. Sometimes, you can get stock options for the company, and you could do well if it makes it public.

I want to say a word about self-confidence here. Many of you are very self-confident, as most doctors are, but some of you may not be. Perhaps you've had some malpractice cases or something adverse happen that shook your confidence. Or, maybe you're confident in your clinical practice but not overall.

I want to tell you that all of you, including you, are incredibly capable. The fact that you've worked so hard in college, medical school, and advanced medical training, and you got where you are regardless of what happened afterward, means that you have tremendous insight, work ethic, and knowledge you could bring to the table.

You may be thinking, "Well, if I'm a consultant or an advisor, or I work for a venture capital firm, what could I offer?" I'm telling you that you could offer a lot. Let's say, for example, you work for a startup. The CEO of that startup is probably brilliant and hardworking as well, but unless they're a physician, they don't have the medical knowledge that you do, no matter how smart they are. You have much to offer these companies; don't ever think you don't.

Imagine you are speaking to your mother, or your brother, or sister, or uncle about a medical topic. Yes, they're probably great people. But unless they're physicians, they don't understand medicine to the depth you do. And beyond that, as physicians, you know how to read studies, understand bias, determine whether something is correlational versus causational, and whether a benefit or risk is significant. You add tremendous value.

You can tease out whether something is anecdotal or something evidence-based. For example, we all hear anecdotally about a terrible tragedy that happened, and it sticks in our minds because it's striking. But if you look at the data, these tragedies may be incredibly rare.

You have the cool head to say, "Well, yes, this is terrible, but this almost never happens." Whereas most people would get caught up in the emotional aspect of the anecdotal story. I say this because even beyond your specialty, you have extraordinary value in how you think about data.

Medical writing. This is another excellent option for clinicians who don't want to be clinicians or for people who lost their medical license or can no longer practice for whatever reason. You could do it from home; you could do it from a boat; you could do it from Europe or Japan. It gives you a lot of flexibility.

What is medical writing? You could, for example, create educational materials about healthcare issues. You could work for a health website. You could work for a pharmaceutical company that wants to produce educational materials about their medication or the disease process they're treating. Hospitals need people to write about diseases and treatments. Insurance companies use writers. Even groups like the VA or other governmental agencies need people to write health educational materials.

You could write about clinical trials. You could summarize them and create reports about them. You could write applications for grants, right? Grants for clinical trials or research. Many people who do research don't want to or know how to write grant applications, and they would be thankful for your help.

As I mentioned earlier, there are a lot of different government jobs where you would write not just educational materials but all aspects of health writing, even health policy writing. You can proofread manuscripts. Many entities produce manuscripts, from researchers to pharmaceutical companies to health insurance companies that write different policies. They need someone to write them and to proofread them.

There's medical communication for marketing agencies. To me, this is kind of a fun one. It is something I would probably be interested in. If you're with a social media marketing company promoting a medically oriented product, they might speak with you to learn more about the disease or its treatment. Your marketing colleagues ask you to proofread the ads or images they've created to see whether they're legit.

If you're one of the more creative types, you could potentially be involved with things like websites, social media content, or slide decks for marketing or advertising agencies in the overall health and wellness sphere.

You could think of it, if you will, as maybe a supplement company that is coming up with some new vitamin product. And they might consult with you about how to advertise it in a way that makes sense medically, or perhaps you'd even create it for them. How fun would that be?

Utilization review. This one is important but probably not as much fun as the marketing stuff, but it certainly would appeal to people who understand how systems should work. The definition that I've seen of utilization review (UR) is that it ensures that patients get the care they need in appropriate settings.

And from what I understand, there are two kinds of angles, if you will, to UR. One is on the hospital or the medical provider side, and the other is on the payer or insurance side.

On the hospital or medical provider side, you'll typically do this. Let's say you have a patient who was in an accident, and they were admitted into the ICU for management. The hospital would have a utilization review team that would, at some interval, check to ensure that it makes sense for this patient to be in the ICU. Perhaps they could be moved to a lower level of care, like a step-down unit or the floor.

Alternatively, although this is probably less common, the UR team would recommend that the patient be sent to a more tertiary or long-term facility that can handle this patient better than you can.

On the other side of the coin, you have insurance companies or payers that also have utilization reviews. They look at things and decide, "Was this justified? Did the patient really need the MRI? Did they need to be on this expensive medication? Do they still need to be in the ICU?" They have tremendous power to determine whether the insurance company will pay.

The way I understand it, the hospital uses UR to protect themselves from the insurance company's UR deciding that what they're doing is inappropriate. For example, the insurance company may not pay for keeping someone in the ICU longer than they feel is necessary. So the hospital's utilization review, in theory, would say, "Hey, this patient needs to leave the ICU and go to the floor," thereby preventing the hospital from keeping someone in the ICU and then only later being told that the insurance company won't pay for it.

It's a bit of a game, but it has a lot of value in that it helps reduce the overall cost of healthcare because people aren't getting unnecessary treatment. And it is likely better for patients because, in theory, you're making sure that patients are getting the level of care they need without going overboard.

I know if I were a patient or a family member were a patient, I wouldn't want to be in the ICU if I didn't need to be. I wouldn't want to get an unnecessary CT scan just because the medical center wanted to bill for a CT scan. Please save me from that!

If you are a clinically practicing physician now, you may have had an adversarial relationship with the utilization review people. But if you were a patient or if you were in charge of the overall healthcare system, you may find that the utilization review team works for your benefit by preventing needless procedures, by preventing some unethical physicians or hospital groups from doing more than is required, and by reducing the overall cost of healthcare in the US. If this appeals to you, UR is a great opportunity. There are many ways to get involved, either through the medical centers or the payers.

All right, now I want to talk about something I have a lot of personal experience with, and I love consulting with my physician clients about this. Let's discuss starting your own business.

I've started several of my own businesses. Some of them were in the medical sphere, and some were not. I had one startup providing telemedicine for athletes, and I created that from scratch. But then I had some other enterprises that were entirely nonmedical.

For example, I started a business where we helped people use virtual or augmented reality to stage homes. That's relatively common now. But when I was starting this, I guess I'll toot my own horn and say it was a bit ahead of its time because not many were using it. Maybe I was too ahead of my time because it didn't work out, but it was a fun experience. I learned a lot from it. I love real estate, and I like technology. It was a great marriage for me. But it was totally nonmedical. It was just something that I was interested in. I had another real estate-related project where I was trying to help seniors find alternative housing types that they could afford, like accessory dwelling units or Golden Girls-style housing. I tell you this just because I want you to realize that the world is your oyster if you want to go and start your own business.

Because you're a physician, the path of least resistance for you would be to do something in healthcare. Perhaps you've even thought about this already. Maybe you've seen a problem you are frustrated by and thought, "Well, why is it done this way? Why do we have to do it this way instead of that way, which would be more efficient?"

If you've identified a problem that needs to be fixed and you come up with a solution, that could be very valuable. And if you've done that in the healthcare space, and it's something you understand well and have had to deal with personally, it may be worth exploring your idea further.

In general, the best businesses identify a legitimate problem that frustrates people or causes harm and then find a solution to that problem.

If you've got that, you're in great shape to develop a good small business idea. And because you are a physician, you automatically have credibility. For example, suppose you've decided to start a small business that is a new patient management system for ambulatory surgery centers. In that case, you have a lot of credibility to do that versus, let's say, some lawyer or some recent college graduate who came up with a similar idea. People are going to trust you more because you know the space. This is beneficial because opening doors and meeting with people about your business will be easier.

If you have a business idea in the medical field and you want to pitch this idea to investors, you have credibility. If you have a healthcare idea but lack programming skills, you have credibility when you pitch to a technical co-founder. They will want to join your business because they'll think, "Well, this person's a physician. They know what they're talking about, and we can make a good team."

Think of the alternative. Let's say you're not a physician, and you've just graduated from business school two or three years ago or graduated college a couple of years ago. You go to the technical co-founder. That person will likely think, "Well, who are you, and what do you bring to the table?" So you won't get as far if you're not a physician.

If you are a physician, tons of people will naturally talk to you, give you credibility, and even give you ethical credibility because there's this presumption that physicians are honorable people. They're more likely to meet with you, and you can go places with your small business if you want to. Being a physician is beneficial in a small business or when starting a business, even if it's not in the healthcare space.

For example, let's say you have an idea to create a new consumer product, or you have an idea in the real estate space. If you go and pitch to investors or potential partners, people are more likely to listen to you because you're a physician, even for most nonmedical topics. But they probably won't give you the same level of credibility as in healthcare.

In other words, let's say you're pitching a real estate product to someone, a startup you've come up with in the real estate space. People will not necessarily assume that you are a real estate expert, but they will assume that you're smart. They will assume that you're ethical. They will assume you are hardworking and know how to get things done.

Imagine pitching a real estate startup versus, say, someone who graduated college a couple of years ago. Unless that person is already a real estate expert, investors are more likely to listen to you. If you try to reach out to someone on Linkedin and have MD after your name, potential contacts are much more likely to speak to you and hear what you have to say. There's a presumption that you are a person of substance versus some random person who may seem shady. So, regardless of whether you're interested in health or another field, physicians like you are well-positioned to launch a small business startup.

Being in a small business or startup has many benefits, including being fun and creative. You use your brain in ways you may not have before. Anyone who's in a small business, at least early on, has to do all kinds of tasks that they might eventually farm out to other people. But as a startup, you need to figure out these things yourself, like marketing and advertising, HR, how you will hire partners or employees, or whether you'll outsource things. You even have to learn some accounting, and you have to learn some basics of the laws that impact small businesses.

With all of these hats, you learn so much. So, if you're the type of person who likes learning new things, starting a business is one of the best ways to do it.

There are disadvantages to being an entrepreneur. Of course, the biggest problem is that the chance of success of any small business is low. So, suppose you're currently a practicing clinician, and you decide to leave clinical practice and start a small business. You'll likely make much less money in the small business than you do in your current clinical career. Even if you make money as an entrepreneur, it will probably be far in the future.

If you start a small business, you need to have a high tolerance for risk. Some companies are insanely successful, but you want to be realistic, especially if you're giving up a lucrative career.

Startups are time-consuming. Yes, you may not have much to do at two or three in the morning. And yes, you probably can sleep in your own bed most nights, but you'll face a lot of hours. And for your small business to be successful, it'll take a lot of work.

So I wouldn't do it if your goal is to work less, because I don't think you'll save work here. You'll change the work. You may not be on call, but you may still have to do stuff on weekends or holidays and have long work weeks. Expect that.

The other thing about small businesses that many physicians may not be used to is networking. To have a successful small business, you will need to meet other people, whether it's investors, co-founders, employees, people that you want to sell your product to, suppliers that you need to buy products from, or distributors. It all depends on your industry. You need to meet other people, and you might be able to do a lot of that online, say on LinkedIn, for example. But you're probably also going to have to do it in person.

For some of you, this will be appealing. For others, it may not be. So, you have to consider whether the business you're thinking of starting matches your networking desires and whether you could step up to the plate for that.

Next is real estate. I love real estate. As I mentioned throughout the book, I've done several real estate projects, including the real estate small businesses I discussed earlier. But I've also bought properties for investment, put renters in them, and held them. I flipped properties where I've upgraded and sold them virtually overnight. And I started a real estate syndicate called Electric Avenue Properties with a fellow physician.

Electric Avenue Properties buys properties near new or upcoming electric vehicle plants. Our presumption is that these homes will significantly appreciate once the plant is built and you have a bunch of high-paid tech-ish workers moving into town.

There are a lot of opportunities in real estate at all levels, and you might just do something relatively simple, like buy an investment property or maybe buy a small building. You could do something more advanced, like real estate syndication or commercial real estate. Or, you might want to do something in health-related real estate. For example, you might want to buy hospitals, build a surgery center, or buy existing medical facilities and run them. There are many ways you can jump in.

I love real estate because, in my opinion, it's much more likely to succeed than starting a small business. It's something that you have some control over. You could do it on your own if you want, or you could do it with partners. If you put time into it, I believe you will master the process. Plus, you own a real, tangible asset.

If you buy an investment property, for example, even if things don't work out, even if it doesn't go up in value the way you hoped it would, you still own a physical asset you could sell. It's not something that will go to zero.

Contrast that with a small business that fails. That business could be worth zero. Look at stocks stocks. Granted, it doesn't happen that often. But you could buy stocks or corporate bonds, and then if the company goes belly up, your portfolio may be worthless. If you own real estate, it still has some value. I'm not a financial planner or an accountant, as I said. So, if you're considering investing, you should speak to a qualified person to advise you. I cannot give you financial advice. I am only sharing with you that there are many options in real estate. You can invest on the side and buy a property here and there. Or, you can go all-out and set up a syndication, manage 50 properties, or run a hospital. There are plenty of options. Find something that suits your needs.

As of the writing of this book in late 2023, interest rates have shot through the roof. That makes real estate at this moment much more complicated than it was in years gone by. Because of the high rates, it's hard to buy properties and finance them profitably. And if rates keep going up, the property markets could hit the skids. Given the economic reality of the times, you'll have to see whether this endeavor makes sense for your goals.

What I mean by that is you might find a house you love, a location you love, or an industry you like. Surgery centers, for example. But if the macroeconomic environment isn't good and we slip into a recession, you're swimming upstream. Something to consider, especially if you're taking out loans. Speak to a financial advisor.

Moving on. There's nonmedical philanthropy. We talked about medical charity earlier, such as missions or Mercy Ships. You could even set up free clinics or volunteer in free clinics.

But there are also nonmedical philanthropic activities you could do if you're tired of the clinic. I've been involved in a couple of these myself. We launched one to help encourage girls to get involved in sports. So, I co-founded this group called From Soccer to C-Suite.

Granted, I'm a little biased here because I have two daughters. The project is based on research that found that girls are more likely to become successful businesswomen as adults when they play youth sports. If you're looking at what kind of intervention we could do now to position our kids for success later, one good way to do it is to get them to play sports.

We had conferences in person and virtually, bringing together many interesting people like athletic directors, women in small business, and teenage girls looking toward their future. And we tried to push them toward playing sports and show them how this is possible and beneficial. You may find something completely different than our From Soccer to C-Suite program. Perhaps you want to help animals, or help veterans, or do anything you want. There are practically limitless opportunities to do philanthropy.

If this is something that interests you, being a physician is beneficial. If you're starting a philanthropic group, you must convince others to work with you. Whether it's people who might invest or donate to what you're doing, co-founders you're looking to partner with, suppliers, office space resources, or whatever you're trying to do. You will have a leg up if you have an MD after your name, even for nonclinical projects. People will listen to you and give you a certain amount of credibility, even in spheres outside of clinical medicine. So, if you're interested in philanthropic work, I say go for it. Don't let the fact that it's nonmedical scare you away.

Malpractice consulting or case review. Here's another good one, which people often consider as either a side gig while practicing medicine or something to do afterward. There are different ways to do this.

Typically, you would review cases for a lawyer and say, "Hey, does this seem like malpractice could have occurred here?" or you get into the weeds of the malpractice case. Let me explain.

The way the case review typically works is, let's say, someone had surgery and had an adverse outcome. That person then goes to a lawyer, and they say, "Look, I just had this adverse outcome. I want to sue the doctor, or sue the hospital, or whomever." Typically, the lawyer will send the case to a medical expert for review because the lawyer wants to see whether a standard was violated.

If you are the reviewer, you may say, "Everything was done right. This was just an unfortunate case of bad luck. Things could be done by the book and still not work out." Or you could look at it and say, "Holy smokes. This is a huge deviation from the standard of care. The patient didn't need this surgery, and now they've suffered this complication." This case review will help determine whether or not the lawyer takes the case and how they pursue it.

Alternatively, the defenders, the malpractice insurance companies or hospitals, use case reviewers to look at an adverse outcome and see whether the party they are defending is at fault. They will then make an informed decision about how to proceed.

Then there's malpractice consulting, where you work with the lawyer when the case goes to trial, either on the plaintiff's or defendant's side. You might be called to write about the case or testify in court.

I haven't done this, but I've looked into it quite a bit. It seems like fun. I've spoken to several physicians, and most of them enjoy it. You get paid well. You don't have to work in the middle of the night, and rarely on weekends or holidays. You can frequently work from home unless you're going to testify in court. And it's a way of using your medical expertise without practicing medicine.

There are some disadvantages. It can be uncomfortable for some doctors to work on the plaintiff's side. In other words, many of us may be uneasy being adversarial with fellow physicians. It's not easy to go and say to another doctor, "You did this wrong." We are trained not to do that and have a certain degree of compassion and empathy for fellow doctors.

The other problem is that it could be hard to become known in this space, and you either get no work at all or don't get enough business to make a living. I wouldn't assume you could just leave medicine, do malpractice consulting full-time, put food on the table, and live happily ever after. You'll probably need to build it up over time as you become known. And I wouldn't have this be your Plan A unless you've already done it and broken into the space.

If you do want to do this, there are ways to market yourself, including certain website aggregators that expert witnesses can go to and make themselves known. Lawyers go to these sites and can find you. You could find other ways of promoting yourself directly to lawyers, hospitals, or insurance companies, but it'll take some self-promotion.

Being on TV. I love this. I've been on TV a lot. I've been live as an in-studio guest talking about health topics. I discussed my sustainable home book, *Dr. Greg's Green Home Makeover*. I wrote it to help parents make their houses more sustainable, healthier, and better for the environment.

I've enjoyed a lot of remote TV appearances as well. I've been on Zoom TV interviews nationwide from the comfort of my home office.

It's fun. It's an excellent opportunity to build your brand and spread the word about projects you're working on. It gives you a lot of credibility to say you've been on TV. And did I say that it's fun?

I would love to be one of these regular TV personalities who is frequently a guest talking about the medical topics of the day. You might like this too.

The thing about being on TV is that while it is a blast, it is creative and exciting, and it gives you credibility benefits, it does not typically pay very much. It may not pay anything. In fact, you might have to pay indirectly to do it. You might need to hire a publicist because they know how to open the doors for this.

I would typically refer my physician clients who want to be on TV to my publicist so they can catch fire and get attention. Without a publicist, it's tough to be a star. And again, it's not something you make money off of except in rare circumstances. It's more something you do because you enjoy doing it.

Finally, there's writing. I've written three books. This one is my fourth. I love to do it. I love to share my ideas. I love to help other people. I wrote a book, *Why Doctors Skip Breakfast*, about fasting and anti-aging medicine. That is a favorite topic for me. I love it. I wrote *Dr. Greg's Green Home Makeover* about sustainable, healthy, green homes, particularly for kids. And there's this book you're reading now to support fellow physicians like you.

And if you want to write a book, eBook, or audiobook, I absolutely support you. Many of the people I work with are interested in being an author. I can show you exactly how it's done.

These days, with the abundance of self-publishing, you don't need a publisher to pick up your book. There are many advantages of self-publishing. It's more nimble, and you can talk about whatever you want. You have complete creative control.

The one thing about writing a book is that it takes a lot of time, effort, and, depending on the book, research. And the other thing to understand is that books typically don't make a profit.

If you want to become a writer, yes, you could make a living as a writer. But it's rare. It's rare. The primary way you could make a living as a writer is if you use the writing to sell other services like a consulting service. You use it for credibility. Think of it almost as a top-notch business card. People give you a certain amount of respect because you've written a book about a topic, and then they may hire you as a consultant, an employee, or whatever. The other way to make a living through writing is to use it to promote speaking.

Speaking is a fun thing to do. Depending on how you do it, you might get paid for the speeches. You can even get paid, depending on how you market yourself, your speaking ability, and what you talk about. Writing a book can help you become a speaker, which could then make you money. So writing a book is great. I love doing it. I recommend it if you don't mind the time and are not expecting to profit directly from the book.

So there you have it. These are some of the top nonclinical ways that physicians like you can go and make money if you're tired of taking care of patients or clinical practice or simply can't do it anymore. I hope some of these options inspire you and resonate with you. And if you want to try something different, give them a shot, or let's give them a shot together.

I've tried not to be too self-promotional in this book, but I just want to take a quick second to thank you for reading. The most important thing for a writer is to have readers, so I thank you from the bottom of my heart. We're nearly at the end, but I've still got a few pearls coming up.

Second, I want to ask a favor. If you found this book helpful, please go to wherever you got it and write a nice 5-star review so other people can find the book and benefit. If you know doctors or healthcare professionals who might improve their lives and careers from this information, please share the book with them.

If you'd like to connect, either for questions or to collaborate, please contact me. Find me on LinkedIn (Gregory Charlop, MD) or my website, www.GregoryCharlopMD.com. I'd be delighted to answer your questions and support the next steps in your career.

Chapter 6

Dr. Greg's Top Tips and FAQ

Top Tips

I'm going to share with you some advice that my dad shared with me and that his dad shared with him so many years ago: live below your means. If you're spending a fortune on an unnecessarily extravagant house or have an unreasonably priced car (or cars), the fixed high costs of the mortgage, property taxes, upkeep, car loans, and recurring expenses can drive you into the ground.

Let me tell you a story. Many of my colleagues back when I was at the major hospital in California wanted to work less. They had kids and wanted to spend time with their families. They wished to work 60% or 80% time, but they couldn't because their costs were so high - even considering their extraordinary incomes. The trouble was that their costs were so high for their house, cars, and kids' private education that they simply couldn't work less even though they wanted to.

They had to spend time away from their kids to generate extra income to afford to put their kids in a fancy house and pricy school. It didn't make much sense to me because the primary goal was to have more family time.

If an expensive home or car keeps you away from your family or forces you to work more than you want, I would rethink whether your actions align with your priorities. It may be worth considering moving. We've moved several times. We moved from the San Francisco Bay Area to Los Angeles, then from Los Angeles to Texas, and now Georgia. You don't necessarily need to do all the crazy shenanigans we did, but you may find it worthwhile to relocate to a lower-cost area if you're in a pricy neighborhood now. Many places have affordable homes that you can buy with a great school district for less money.

You might want to consider locales with lower state or property taxes. The cost of gas and groceries varies across the country. Sometimes, the money you save from the move, keeping everything else constant, may allow you to afford a lifestyle similar to what you have now while working less. Different areas also pay different amounts of money, and you'll want to research that when considering if and when to relocate.

Now, we want to review your expenses. Consider costs like taxes, including your state taxes, property taxes, and inheritance taxes, if you're counting on either getting money from family members or giving money to family members. Research how pensions are taxed and distributed. If you're lucky enough to have a pension, you may find it better to avoid specific locations because of their tax burden. Again, I'm not an accountant or a financial planner, so you want to speak to a financial professional.

Next is something we touched on before, but I think it's worth emphasizing here. Think about your financial needs. Explore how and when you want to retire, how long you think you'll live, and how many years of retirement you need to fund.

Where will you live in retirement? What will you do for medical care when you are retired? What will you do if you need nursing care or some other kind of assistance? Will you need to take care of a spouse? What will happen if you are disabled or if your spouse is disabled? Your kids need their costs covered. You may need to pay for their college and grad school. Or, if your kids have special needs, how will you address that now and after you pass on? And you want to think about unplanned costs. We don't know what those will be or when, but we know they will happen. So save some dough for a roof replacement, a new air conditioning system, or a fresh car. You might need money saved up if your job doesn't go the way you wish it to.

Next, I want you to take some time and be philosophical about what you want in life. What makes you happy or unhappy? Where do you find joy? Do you need a radical overhaul of your life, perhaps in a different city? Do you need a job overhaul? Should you retire altogether? Or are you good with something more subtle? Will more free time, an exciting hobby, or a new schedule make you happy? How much of a change do you really need? No one knows that better than you, and you need to think it over.

Next, I want you to think about this question. I ask it of all my physician clients. What is the worst that can happen if you leave your job or leave medicine altogether?

Let's do a thought experiment. Imagine that you decide you don't want to do clinical medicine anymore. Further, pretend you've burned your bridge and cannot return to clinical practice. What's the worst that could happen? Can you adapt? How bad (or good) would it be?

For most people, the worst that could happen isn't so bad. You almost assuredly can get some other type of job, whether it's with a pharmaceutical company, in research, or any number of industries looking to hire physicians. You might even have enough saved up already that you could retire now and enjoy a life of leisure!

Naturally, one way to mitigate your downside risk is to maintain your medical license. That's why I recommend renewing your medical license and CME, which isn't too difficult. Plus, you may get a tax deduction.

And if you can, try to do a small amount of clinical work just to keep your foot in the door and sustain your skills. So, if you're thinking about leaving clinical medicine, I wouldn't give up your license unless you're sure you don't want to go back or you can't go back.

Let me give you an example. I consulted with an urgent care physician preparing to leave medicine because he wanted to devote full-time to his health technology startup. It was a software product that helped patients manage their care. I thought it was a great product, but as with all startups, the chance of success is not that high. He was exploring leaving his clinical practice altogether. We discussed it, and I strongly recommended that he keep his foot in the door instead of abandoning his urgent care practice. Plus, he was fortunate to do urgent care because that's a specialty one can easily do here and there. Demand is high, and you don't have to have a panel of patients to maintain.

We decided that the best thing for him to do would be to almost leave urgent care. He would still do weekend shifts once or twice a month just to maintain his skills and to keep his options open. That way, if he had to return to urgent care if the startup didn't work out, he would be more comfortable and more likely to be hired. Many places are reluctant to employ people in clinical medicine if they haven't worked for a while.

You don't want to be nervous or lose your skills. And you don't want to scare away potential employers.

My next tip is to read the books *The 4-Hour Workweek* and *Die with Zero*. I know I've mentioned these two books before, but it's worth repeating.

The 4-Hour Workweek was the book that gave me permission to work less and to consider my lifestyle, or as Tim Ferriss calls it, lifestyle design, in my decision about how to work, when to work, and how to spend time with family. As odd as it sounds, I needed a book to tell me that it was okay to live my life in the best way for me and my family and friends.

And *Die with Zero* was a powerful reminder that, number one, many of us "over save," which causes us, in effect, to work for nothing. And number two, many of us put off what we want to do until we can no longer do it. Tragic. So do what you can now while you can. Don't have the treadmill mindset, as I call it, where you're putting everything off until you retire.

So, if there is something you really want to do, whether it's backpacking across South America, spending a year living in the United Kingdom, having an RV adventure with your daughter or your spouse, starting a charity, experiencing a remote yoga retreat, training for an ultra marathon, or learning to fly - do it now. Don't wait until after retirement because there is no guarantee that you will have the strength or health. You never know if your future life will throw a wrench in your plans. So do what you really want to do when you can because you may miss your window may close.

My next tip, of course, is to contact me with any questions. I'm always happy to help you elevate your clinical practice or review the pros and cons of exiting clinical medicine entirely. We will use tools to help you determine where you're going, what you want out of life, and how to bring more joy to your clinical or nonclinical practice.

Next, I recommend browsing job sites to get a handle on what's out there. You can find nonclinical jobs on Indeed or Glassdoor. LinkedIn also has a great tool to find employment. You always want to know your worth and understand your options. If you're kicking the tires on a new career, check out the job sites and see what else is in your area (or wherever you want to live). You will get a sense of the job requirements, where you'd have to live, and how much you'd get paid. You might even want to take it a step further and contact some of these jobs, speak to the recruiters, and find out more about them.

Explore job websites for your medical specialty. In anesthesia, for example, GasWork is a great resource to find W2 and 1099 opportunities. There are websites like that for most medical specialties. Find the one that's appropriate for you. Look for jobs that are full-time or part-time. Look for jobs that are near you or in a different state altogether. Look at what's out there to get a sense of your worth because the truth is, unless you start looking at other options, you never really know where you stand. In other words, you might be significantly underpaid and overworked compared to the industry norm.

Or the opposite might be true. You might have a pretty sweet gig and not realize it until you see what else exists.

Finally, when looking at other medical job opportunities, you may have to do some digging for certain universities, the VA, and specific small and large medical centers. You might find that information only on particular websites. And freelancing opportunities sometimes can only be found in certain places online. I love to work on this with my clients. But if you're doing this on your own, spend some time; look and see what the different websites are; see what else is out there. Another way to explore the job market is to go directly to locum companies appropriate for your specialty.

If you're an emergency medicine doctor or an internist, you can find locum companies that work with your niche. Go to their websites and look at the available jobs. Again, you may not take any of them, but at least you can learn what opportunities exist across the country, how much they pay, what the job expectations are, and whether some of them might offer a lifestyle that's better or worse than the one you have right now.

Another tip, and this isn't fun, but I think you have to do it, is to start working on your resume. I tell you from personal experience that I didn't like doing this, and most people don't particularly enjoy working on their resume because you have to pull together dates and locations and everything else. But the benefit is that you have a resume (or CV) ready to go that you could deploy the moment you find an intriguing opportunity. You might even want to make two resumes, one for clinical positions and the other for non-medical jobs.

For your clinical resume or CV, make sure you have details about all your various medical accomplishments, your different titles, the committees you've served on, research, and that type of thing. Include specific medical skills, such as ultrasound use or acupuncture. Your nonclinical resume will focus more on outside projects, books you've written, businesses you've started, and courses you've taken outside medicine. For example, include your startup consulting work or that class you took last summer on accounting.

Make friends in other industries. If you are considering going into management consulting, or you want to become a medical writer, or you want to become an investment banker, or perhaps you want to become a lawyer, for example, I would recommend that you go out and make friends who do the very thing you're looking to do. You remember back in the day before you went to medical school, everybody said, "You know what? You should volunteer at a hospital or a clinic to see what it's like to do medicine." Well, the same is true if you want to go into one of these other fields.

If you're thinking about becoming an investment banker, go out, meet some investment bankers, and chat with them to see what their life is like. You might love it, you might not. Remember, the grass isn't always greener on the other side of the fence, but sometimes it is. And as far as how to do this, one of my favorite ways is LinkedIn. I love meeting people on LinkedIn. In fact, you can connect with me, Gregory Charlop. Say hi! Be sure to look for people in the specialties or fields you're considering and make friends with them. Invite them to coffee or virtual coffee and discover what life is like in their world. What do they like, and what don't they like about their lifestyle?

My final tip, which should go without saying, but I will say it anyway, is to speak with your loved ones. Your loved ones care about you; they have your best interest and heart; they've seen what makes you happy and what makes you unhappy. Try to get their opinion. You don't necessarily need to follow it, but it's good to hear them out. If you have childhood or lifelong friends, ask them. Bounce ideas off them. And most importantly, if you have a spouse, find out how they feel about your situation. Ask, "Would you be willing to move? How would you feel if I made less money but switched jobs? Are you willing to take the financial uncertainty of me leaving my current secure job for something else? Are you happy with the way things are now or not?" And I'll tell you, you might find out that your spouse is just as unhappy as you are, and they may be thrilled with the opportunity of moving.

Conversely, if your spouse is taking care of their sick mother, the idea of moving may be unacceptable. You must find this stuff out before you get too into the weeds about moving or radical lifestyle overhauls.

Frequently Asked Questions

Question one:

Can I get back into medicine if I leave? I get this question all the time. And the answer, to quote a radiologist, is, "It depends." Typically, the answer is yes. As long as you haven't been gone for too long, you haven't let your medical licenses expire, and you have maintained some exposure to clinical practice and your CME credits, it isn't too difficult to return to clinical medicine if you choose. You may find it's easier than you think because, with the doctor shortage, most places would be delighted to have you back. It depends on how long you've been out, what's happened to your medical licenses or malpractice insurance, your specialty, and if you performed any clinical practice in the last two years.

When you think about whether you can return to medicine if you leave, there are two issues to consider. Number One, are you comfortable and competent to do it? Do you still have your skills, and are you not freaked out about the idea? And Number Two, will someone hire you? In most cases, if you want to restart a clinical practice, you can. So, to answer the earlier question: What's the worst that can happen if you leave? Probably not much.

Question two:

I care for tertiary patients at high-level hospitals. What happens if I stop taking care of those patients? Great question. A couple of things could happen. You might leave and decide you never want to deal with those patients again. With some space, you might discover that you were doing it just because you *were* doing it (treadmill), and now you're happier without the aggravation. Alternatively, you might leave and then realize that you loved the tertiary patients and decide to go back.

My sense is if that's how you feel, you'll figure that out pretty quickly. If you move fast, you won't lose any skills, and you'll have plenty of opportunities to return. But most doctors find that they're okay with "routine" patients.

Let me give you an anesthesia example. Let's say that after completing your cardiac anesthesia fellowship, you spent most of your time with patients with end-stage heart disease undergoing major operations. You became accustomed to that population. Even though you know cognitively this isn't true, viscerally, you felt every patient suffered from a low ejection fraction. But the truth is that most people undergoing surgery are ordinary, relatively healthy folks undergoing routine procedures.

If you left that tertiary world and no longer took care of seniors with heart transplants, even if you lost the ability or the desire to do that, you'll find that there are tons of other ways you could work in the OR. Because the vast majority of folks, as I said, are getting regular things done like tonsillectomies or knee scopes.

The same is true in any specialty. If you work in urgent care at a major academic center, you're used to taking care of elderly patients with severe COPD and chest pain. If you leave and go to a local community facility, you'll find that most people come in with headaches or sore throats. There are all kinds of urgent care. There are many ways you can help patients, and most of them are not tertiary. So don't worry about it. You'll find a job, and I think you'll be just as happy, if not happier.

Question three:

What team do I need if I switch jobs or leave medicine? If you decide to depart a stable W2 medical job, you'll definitely want some professionals by your side. You'll want an accountant to ensure you're doing your taxes. Your taxes as a freelancer or entrepreneur can be more complex than you're used to. You need someone to keep an eagle eye on you to let you know whether you're spending too much or too little.

I would have a financial planner. I recommend all my clients at least meet initially with a financial planner to see where they stand, how much of a cushion they have, and whether they could switch careers or take a financial hit and be fine. It helps to have an ongoing relationship with one to help manage your retirement accounts.

Before you leave your current job, I recommend you retain a lawyer to review your contract to evaluate whether you have any restrictions. A lawyer will also examine your new contracts before you sign. Please ensure you're not signing something that could put you at risk. For example, be careful with non-compete arrangements.

You want an insurance broker for malpractice insurance since if you continue clinical practice, you'll need a policy. I advise retaining a broker for your other insurance policies, like life, disability, and car.

Question four:

Do you recommend freelancing to everyone? No. That may surprise you since I do it, and I love it, and I recommend it to many people, but I certainly don't recommend it to *all* people. Folks with a very low risk tolerance will struggle freelancing because there's no guarantee that your company or the group will need you tomorrow. Any opportunity could dry up, and you could be out of luck.

If you have trouble managing your finances and require handholding, freelancing may not be a good idea. You know what I mean. I know you're an intelligent, creative, driven person. You did all these things to get into medical school. But if you don't like managing your 401(k)s, pensions, retirement plans, and following up on how much you need to save or what stocks to own, and you're not good about managing all your insurance policies and everything else, a W2 job may be better for you.

Because the truth is, if you're working independently, at the end of the day, you have to keep an eye on all that, and some people just don't like to do it. Some find it an irritation and just don't want that responsibility. So, If that's you, stay at a W2 job or find a financial professional you trust who will do everything for you.

Another reason freelancing may not make sense is if you live in an area without many freelancing opportunities and are unable or unwilling to move.

I'll give you a personal example. As I mentioned, we moved just outside Austin, Texas, for a year. I didn't do my research before going. That was another one of life's lessons. It turns out that particular area is not very good for anesthesia freelancing.

Most anesthesia care was run by a few groups, many owned by private equity firms. It was difficult for me to find the freelancing jobs I was looking for. They were there, but there weren't many of them, and they required a lot of travel. As of this writing, other places like Dallas, for example, had ample freelancing opportunities. Austin, not so much. If this is not an easy option where you live, it may not work for you, or you might have to move. Go to your medical specialty job site. This will help you evaluate freelancing opportunities where you live.

Finally, freelancing may not be appropriate for you if you are not flexible. You've got to be honest with yourself. In my old job, some people had to have everything a certain way. They required the patient to be brought into the operating room in a certain way. They could only use one type of IV catheter; nothing else was safe. They could only use one kind of tubing. Everything had to be just how they liked it, or else it was "unsafe." At least, that's how they felt. They were able to mold their practice to fit their preferences, which is fine; more power to them. But someone like that would have difficulty freelancing in different centers. If you're walking in the door somewhere with an existing practice and filling in for a day, a week, or three times a month, you must go with the flow. You will not be able to remake that practice in your image.

If you're cool with that and think freelancing will be exciting because you learn different ways to work, then go for it. This might be a plus for you. But if you're not cool with that, if you're not that flexible or open-minded to different things, and I need you to be honest here with me and with yourself, then perhaps jumping from job to job is just not going to suit your personality.

Question five:

Should I leave medicine if I want to make more money? I would say no. Now, I support people looking to make more money. I'm all for making money. It's great. But as I mentioned earlier, medicine, on average, is one of the highest-paying fields. It's unlikely, but not impossible, to generate more revenue from another profession. Anything can happen, but I wouldn't count on it.

You may be able to make more money in medicine than you are today by switching cities or states. Some places pay more or have lower taxes. Food and gas are cheaper in some states than others. You can try to renegotiate a better contract with your existing group or move to a more lucrative medical practice. Just understand that you're unlikely to make more money out of medicine unless you hit a home run.

Last Question:

How can you and I work together? I'm glad you asked! I'm happy to work with you. My group, the Physician Wellness Project, helps physicians like you improve your work-life balance and experience more joy in your career. I'm honored to support you. You can connect with me on my website, www.GregoryCharlopMD.com, Gregory Charlop on LinkedIn, or look for the Physician Wellness Project.

I love doing one-on-one consultations, and we are finalizing some remarkable online courses to learn at your own pace with complete privacy. You'll learn:

- How to determine why you're unhappy with your current job

- How to take a clear-eyed look at your financial situation

- How to increase your joy in clinical practice, or how to move beyond medicine

- How to escape the traps and find happiness, fulfillment, and more time for your health, family, friends, loved ones, and hobbies

Let's work together to help you live your best life. Learn more at www.GregoryCharlopMD.com.

Chapter 7

Conclusion

You were four years old. Your friends were out having a good time climbing trees, playing tag, and doing all the stuff that children do. You were inside practicing the violin. Ever since you were little, you've spent your days learning or training instead of being a kid. Why? Because you were on the launching pad to be a physician.

The long runway required to become a doctor involves years of hard work and sacrifice. From a young age, you had to give up splashing in muddy puddles, going to high school parties, and experiencing once-in-a-lifetime college adventures because you were studying, working on extracurricular activities, or trying to change the world. All this to get into medical school.

You're a doctor now, but life didn't turn out as you expected. Your tastes changed. You feel burnt out and suffer from moral injury because every effort you make to help patients is thwarted by administration or bureaucracy. Perhaps you are physically unable to take call or work nights. Or, you've prioritized your children and family over your medical practice. Work isn't working out.

You've given up so much to get where you are, and you deserve the best. After all your sacrifices, you deserve a life that matches your dreams.

Your friends and family care about you; they want you to be happy, and they know you put in a lot of sweat and tears to get where you are. But unfortunately, most people outside of medicine simply don't understand what you've gone through. Most folks don't realize the sacrifices you made since you were a toddler. They don't know what it is like to be on call. They don't know what it is like to work in an ICU and see a sick patient slip away. They can't possibly know because they've never experienced it.

While they certainly wish you the best, they don't know what it's like. Only other physicians do. And so I'm telling you, one physician to another, give yourself permission to be happy. Give yourself permission to reconfigure your life to experience joy and meaning.

That is my mission. I stand with you. The Physician Wellness Project aims to help all doctors rekindle their joy. Let's collaborate to bring your life more meaning and balance.

But even without me, you can do all of this on your own as long as you give yourself permission to be open-minded and do your research. Go out there, open your eyes, and see what you can do. You only have one life to live - live it well.

If you found this book helpful, please do me a favor. Like you, I am a physician striving to help others. Please write a nice five-star review wherever you got this book, and share the book with anyone that you think might benefit.

Together, we can start a movement to make healthcare better for everybody. And if you'd like more information, I'm constantly posting free, valuable videos on my YouTube channel or my website, www.GregoryCharlopMD.com.

Thank you so much for reading. You've helped my dreams come true, and I wish nothing but the best for you.

ABOUT THE AUTHOR

Gregory Charlop, MD

Physician and father of two daughters, Dr. Gregory Charlop (aka Dr. Greg), is passionate about helping healthcare professionals find joy and meaning in their careers. Since training at Stanford and UCLA, Dr. Greg has become a sought-after speaker, consultant, and nationally recognized medical expert. Dr. Greg is regularly featured on major media outlets, including ABC, NBC, CBS, Forbes, and FOX.

He founded the Physician Wellness Project, which tackles physician and nurse burnout. He offers one-on-one consulting and online courses to help doctors and nurses improve their careers and work-life balance.

Philanthropy is at the core of Dr. Greg's work. He allied with leading charities and social-impact investors to create From Soccer to C-Suite™, a multi-state leadership conference. His events support children's mental health and minority women entrepreneurs.

He founded the Women's Sports Forum series of conferences, podcasts, and events featuring powerful women athletes and business executives. He aims to inspire young girls to become leaders by sharing the stories of successful women.

Dr. Greg co-founded Electric Avenue Properties LLC, a syndicate that invests in sustainable properties near newly announced electric vehicle and battery plants in Georgia and Ohio. His team supports community development to encourage the adoption of green transit and housing.

Concerned with global health and prosperity, Dr. Greg and his team are organizing an invite-only international consortium of business and thought leaders. The group promotes multinational networking and understanding.

The Physician Wellness Project is Dr. Greg's fourth book. His earlier titles include Dr. Greg's Green Home Makeover: Your Family's Guide to Healthy, Sustainable Living and Why Doctors Skip Breakfast: Wellness Tips to Reverse Aging, Treat Depression, and Get a Good Night's Sleep. His writing focuses on how humans and the planet can stay healthy and thrive.

If you're a doctor or nurse looking to improve your career and consult with Dr. Greg, please reach out at www.GregoryCharlopMD.com. He's also available to hospitals and health organizations for speaking and consulting.

www.ingramcontent.com/pod-product-compliance
Lightning Source LLC
Chambersburg PA
CBHW060326130626
46553CB00003B/932